# ~~TAKE~~ *Eat* YOUR VITAMINS

Your Guide to Using Natural Foods to Get the Vitamins, Minerals, and Nutrients *Your Body Needs*

## Mascha Davis, MPH, RDN

ADAMS MEDIA

New York   London   Toronto   Sydney   New Delhi

*To JD—*
*Thank you for the endless laughter, support, and inspiration.*

---

*Special acknowledgment and thanks to Paula Szwedowski for
her assistance in researching and writing this book.*

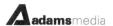

Adams Media
An Imprint of Simon & Schuster, LLC
100 Technology Center Drive
Stoughton, MA 02072

Copyright © 2020 by Simon & Schuster, LLC

All rights reserved, including the right to reproduce
this book or portions thereof in any form whatsoever.
For information address Adams Media Subsidiary
Rights Department, 1230 Avenue of the Americas,
New York, NY 10020.

First Adams Media trade paperback edition
January 2020

ADAMS MEDIA and colophon are trademarks of
Simon & Schuster.

For information about special discounts for bulk
purchases, please contact Simon & Schuster
Special Sales at 1-866-506-1949 or business@
simonandschuster.com.

The Simon & Schuster Speakers Bureau can bring
authors to your live event. For more information or to
book an event contact the Simon & Schuster Speakers
Bureau at 1-866-248-3049 or visit our website at
www.simonspeakers.com.

Interior design by Colleen Cunningham and
Priscilla Yuen
Interior image © 123RF

Manufactured in the United States of America

6 2023

Library of Congress Cataloging-in-Publication Data
Names: Davis, Mascha, author.
Title: Eat your vitamins / Mascha Davis, MPH, RDN.
Description: Avon, Massachusetts: Adams Media, 2020.
Includes index.
Identifiers: LCCN 2019039416 | ISBN 9781507211359
(pb) | ISBN 9781507211342 (ebook)
Subjects: LCSH: Cooking (Natural foods) | Nutrition. |
Natural foods. | Functional foods. | LCGFT: Cookbooks.
Classification: LCC TX741 .D3877 2020 |
DDC 641.3/02--dc23
LC record available at
https://lccn.loc.gov/2019039416

ISBN 978-1-5072-1135-9
ISBN 978-1-5072-1134-2 (ebook)

# Contents

## Introduction 5

## Why Eat Your Vitamins? 6

# Final Thoughts

# US/Metric Conversion Charts

# Index

# Introduction

- Looking to boost your $B_{12}$? Try some clams.
- Need more niacin? Have some turkey.
- Craving more calcium? Try some fresh greens.

Want your body to function to its fullest potential with all its vitamin and nutrient needs met? Then the solution you're searching for doesn't come in a pill bottle; it comes from real, natural food. Why? Your body is built to optimally utilize nutrients from *real* food, rather than in synthetic or processed forms. But each year people spend an astounding $30 billion on powdered supplements and pills. Something isn't quite adding up.

In *Eat Your Vitamins*, you'll learn exactly what vitamins, minerals, and nutrients you need, how much you should be consuming, and how and why you should be getting them from natural foods—rather than from costly supplements or processed compounds in a bottle. To make it easy, this book is divided into over forty entries, each focused on a particular nutrient. Inside you'll find all the info you need to start meeting your dietary needs and improving your health immediately, including:

- Benefits of each nutrient
- What effects it can have on your body
- Some precautions and warnings
- Recommended amounts for different age groups
- The best natural foods for obtaining the nutrient
- A delicious recipe to help you gain all that nutrient's benefits in a *natural* way

There is no shortcut to good health, but there are some simple practices that you can easily incorporate into your lifestyle, no matter how busy you are. This book is your guide to nourishing your body, optimizing your well-being, and, best of all, getting the nutrients and vitamins your body needs by eating delicious (and real) food!

# Why Eat Your Vitamins?

The term "vitamin" originates from the term *vital amines*, meaning "essential to life." Most natural, minimally processed foods are bursting with vitamins, minerals, and nutrients. For example, a serving each of berries, snap peas, and greens provides enough vitamin C, folate, and potassium to almost meet the average adult's daily requirements. Whole grains are full of fiber and prebiotics to feed your gut flora, B-complex vitamins give you the energy you need, and fish has the omega-3s to reduce inflammation in your body. When you understand which foods have the nutrients you require and how much you actually need, you can then understand how to plan your diet in a way that ensures you are getting the vitamins and minerals essential to your health and not just guessing—or hoping—that a supplemental pill or powder might make up for what you are missing. In short, the best way to get more energy, a stronger immune system, glowing skin, and overall better health is through the foods you eat, not the pills you take.

## Supplements Aren't the Answer

According to top nutrition experts at Harvard Medical School, as well as numerous research studies, most nutrients are better absorbed and used by the body when consumed from a whole food instead of a supplement. However, many people feel the need to take pills, powders, and supplements in an attempt to obtain nutrients and fill the gaps in their diets. We hope these will give us more energy, prevent us from catching a cold in the winter, or improve our skin and hair. But in reality, the large majority of supplements are synthetic and unregulated, and may not even be completely absorbed by your body. Worse, some are contaminated with other substances and contain ingredients not listed on the label. For example, a recent investigative report found heavy metals in 40 percent of 134 brands of protein powders on the market. With little oversight and regulation, taking supplements is a gamble and often expensive. It should only be done with caution and the guidance of a dietitian.

And vitamins are not the only nutrients we feel we need to supplement with pills or powders. We take protein powder instead of eating protein-rich foods; we take antioxidant pills when the antioxidant power of some berries and fruits is far beyond what most pills contain. The multibillion-dollar supplement industry has capitalized on people's desire to be healthy and to find that "silver bullet" that will cure their ills or help to heal their health problems. The truth is, taking supplements is often unnecessary, and it can even be harmful.

There are, of course, exceptions to every rule, and there are definitely cases when supplementation is needed and can be beneficial, such as with specific medical conditions, for a clinical deficiency (measured by a lab result), during pregnancy when nutritional needs greatly increase, and even for some nutrients that are difficult to get from food sources, like vitamin D. To safely use supplements, be sure to talk with your doctor and make an appointment with a registered dietitian before you begin any dietary changes.

## Better Health Through Food

You've likely heard the classic phrase "Let food be thy medicine," attributed to the ancient Greek physician Hippocrates around 400 B.C. Since early times, civilizations have observed the powerful, nurturing, and healing effects of the foods that we eat. Many of the illnesses we face today have their root causes in lack of proper nutrition. But it's no wonder that so many people are confused about what, when, and how to eat. With the explosion of social media and the click-bait news cycle that we live in, misinformation or misrepresentation of information is rampant. Many spokespeople or influencers who never studied nutrition or health are able to promote products and diets to a wide audience. News outlets, desperate for eyeballs and clicks, publish sensationalistic headlines that misrepresent the actual research in order to get people to look at them. And it works! Quick fixes, extreme diets, and the "silver bullet" solutions are really tempting. Often, they are presented in such a convincing way that anyone who *isn't* an expert would be confused as to whether to believe it or not.

When you take the time to slow down, learn about how to nourish yourself with whole foods, and observe how you feel, you can change your health and your life. The way you approach food and your relationship to your body and nutrition are also incredibly important. This shift requires gaining some knowledge from credible sources, incorporating fewer processed items, and giving yourself permission to explore and enjoy a wide variety of whole foods.

After all, the current normal isn't working. Many people have been sold on diets defined by processed, nutrient-poor fast food; added sugars and sodas; refined grains; and few fresh fruits and vegetables. Others have almost cut out entire food groups, such as carbohydrates, while others are still avoiding healthful foods like fats. These unbalanced ways of eating can cause you to miss many of the essential, life-giving nutrients, leading to skyrocketing rates of chronic disease, inflammation, nutrient deficiencies, and obesity. But there's a way to shift this, and it begins with an understanding of what your body needs to function at its best.

Your body needs certain nutrients and vitamins to survive and thrive, so why can't you just swallow a pill that contains those particular nutrients? It is best for your body and your overall health to get these nutrients from food sources. Why?

- Food sources are more bioavailable (better absorbed by the body).
- Foods come as part of a nutrient-dense package that has many more benefits than the nutrient alone, in isolation. For example, not only do fruits have vitamin C; they also come with a whole package of other nutrients like prebiotics, polyphenols, and potassium, to name just a few. These nutrients often work together symbiotically and boost the action or bioavailability of one another.
- Whole foods contain many nutrients and compounds that haven't yet been identified by scientists, but we know they have many positive effects. What makes whole foods so healthy is the synergy of these nutrients, and how they work together, rather than single, isolated compounds.

With that in mind, we will explore over forty nutrients, each in its own easy-to-read section, with a description; an overview of its roles in the body and benefits; and, most important, which foods are highest in the nutrient. You'll also find some precautions and warnings for groups of people with preexisting medical conditions that could interfere with the consumption of the nutrient.

## Try Nutrigenomics

If you want to get specific and personalized recommendations for your body, I recommend that you speak to a dietitian and do a nutrigenomics test. Nutrigenomics is the field of study that looks at genetics and nutrition. There are genetic variants that affect how your body metabolizes different nutrients, including carbs, protein, and fat; your ability to absorb and utilize vitamins; and much more. For example, while we all need carbs, the exact amount varies from person to person. Some people are genetically predisposed to function better on a lower carb amount, around one third of their plate. Others need as much as half of their plate to consist of carbohydrate-rich foods to meet their needs and optimize their health. Nutrigenomics can also show if you are predisposed to being lower in certain vitamins, which can help to guide lab testing and food selection.

# Vitamin A

If vitamins could confer superpowers, vitamin A would be known for giving you powerful vision; a strong immune system to fight off invaders; and beautiful skin, hair, and nails. This essential nutrient is frequently misunderstood, and there's a lot of confusion about its various forms, benefits, dangers, and uses. Most people in the US get plenty of this vitamin from their diets, but, sadly, vitamin A deficiency is the main cause of blindness in developing countries. It's ideal to get vitamin A entirely from food sources, such as eggs, fish, spinach, and carrots, as well as many others that you will learn about in this entry.

## Description

Vitamin A helps boost immunity, keeps your eyes healthy, and ensures that your reproductive system functions properly. It's also an antioxidant, which means it can help fight harmful compounds called free radicals.

There are two main forms of vitamin A that you can get from food:

- **Active vitamin A:** This is fully formed and found only in animal-based products. The body can use this form right away as well as store it. It is made up of a group of compounds called retinoids. Retinoids have many different names, such as retinol, retinal, retinoic acid, and retinyl esters.
- **Pro-vitamin A:** This type of vitamin A is not yet active in the body, but once it is eaten, it gets converted into active vitamin A in your tissues. This form is found in fruits and vegetables and is made up of a group of compounds called carotenoids. The most well-known carotenoid is beta-carotene, which is also a pigment that gives many fruits and veggies their bright colors.

Like other fat-soluble vitamins, vitamin A is stored in your body. This vitamin is mainly kept in the liver. When there's a need for extra vitamin A, it's discharged from the liver and travels to where it is needed.

Vitamin A is better absorbed when consumed with a fat. Also, beta-carotene in plants is absorbed more easily when the food is finely chopped or gently cooked, as this helps it to become more bioavailable through the tough cell wall.

## Role in the Body

- **Supports normal heart, kidney, and lung function:** Vitamin A helps make sure that the cells of these essential organs are replicating properly and also participates in their repair.

- **Eye health:** Vitamin A is a component of the proteins that absorb light in the retina and keep your eyes healthy as they develop and as they age.
- **Immune health and cellular communication:** Vitamin A is necessary for different kinds of immune cells to find their proper location and then communicate with other cells so they can take action against invaders like pathogens and bacteria.

## Benefits

- **Reduces inflammation:** Vitamin A is both a vitamin and an antioxidant. It can support the body by reducing the inflammatory process when it's at optimal amounts.
- **Contributes to cell growth:** Vitamin A is necessary for the proper growth and division of cells. This also means that it plays a role in preventing cancer, which is essentially cells receiving the wrong signals and growing out of control.
- **Improves skin health:** While the exact mechanism isn't fully understood, it seems that having the right amount of vitamin A can help prevent acne in some people. It's also important for slowing down ultraviolet

damage from the sun, which causes wrinkles and aging of the skin.

- **Contributes to eye health:** Eating vitamin A–rich foods helps to keep your eyes healthy as you age, possibly because of its antioxidant effects and the fact that vitamin A produces the main pigments of your eyes.
- **Helps to prevent cancer:** Studies have shown that consuming beta-carotene obtained from plants can help to prevent cancer. Interestingly, this effect is not shown for beta-carotene supplements.

## Side Effects, Warnings, and Precautions

Active vitamin A is not quickly cleared from the body because it is a fat-soluble vitamin. This means that excess vitamin A builds up in fatty tissues. A chronic high intake of active vitamin A can turn the eyes and skin yellow. You can be at risk if you're consuming a lot of foods high in active vitamin A, like liver, or taking high-dose supplements with active vitamin A. It's important to get just the right amount of vitamin A, not too much and not too little. Too much can negate some of the beneficial effects of this amazing vitamin.

## Signs of Deficiency

Vitamin A deficiency is uncommon in most developed nations. Some signs of mild deficiency can include dry skin or dry eyes. Eventually, vitamin A deficiency can lead to blindness, infertility, or delayed growth, but this level of severity is usually only seen in less developed parts of the world. Tragically, up to 500,000 malnourished children in the developing world lose their sight each year due to lack of vitamin A.

## How Much You Need

Amounts of vitamin A are measured in retinol activity equivalents (RAEs) because of the varying levels of bioactivity (how they work in the body) of the different kinds of vitamin A (e.g., retinol versus carotenoids). Here are conversions for RAEs to other common measures of vitamin A:

- 1 RAE = 0.001mg of retinol
- 1 RAE = 0.006mg of beta-carotene
- 1 RAE = 3.3 international units (IUs) of vitamin A

The Food and Drug Administration (FDA) is putting new labeling rules into effect in 2020–2021, stating that vitamin A amounts will be expressed in RAEs instead of IUs. Here are the most recent, updated reference ranges (amounts are per day):

| AGE | MALE | FEMALE |
| --- | --- | --- |
| 0–6 months | 400mcg RAE | 400mcg RAE |
| 7–12 months | 500mcg RAE | 500mcg RAE |
| 1–3 years | 300mcg RAE | 300mcg RAE |
| 4–8 years | 400mcg RAE | 400mcg RAE |
| 9–13 years | 600mcg RAE | 600mcg RAE |
| 14–18 years | 900mcg RAE | 900mcg RAE |
| 19+ years | 900mcg RAE | 700mcg RAE |
| 70+ years | 900mcg RAE | 700mcg RAE |
| Pregnancy | – | 770mcg RAE |
| Lactation | – | 1,300mcg RAE |

## Tolerable Upper Levels

| AGE | AMOUNT PER DAY |
| --- | --- |
| 0–12 months | 600mcg |
| 1–3 years | 600mcg |
| 4–8 years | 900mcg |
| 9–13 years | 1,700mcg |
| 14–18 years | 2,800mcg |
| 19+ | 3,000mcg |

## Best Way to Consume

Vitamin A is plentiful in many foods that are widely available—from eggs and canned fish to many different vegetables and fruits, so the vast majority of people don't need to take a supplement, as long as their meals are balanced.

## Natural Food Sources

Animal-based sources include:

| FOOD (SERVING) | VITAMIN A (MCG RAE) |
| --- | --- |
| Liver, beef (3 ounces) | 6,600 |
| Herring, pickled (3 ounces) | 220 |
| Milk, whole (1 cup) | 150 |
| Egg (1 large) | 75 |
| Cheese (1 ounce) | 60–85 |
| Sardines (3 ounces) | 92 |
| Tuna (3 ounces) | 55 |
| Herring oil (1 tablespoon) | 13.6 |
| Cod liver oil (1 tablespoon) | 13.5 |

Some vegan sources include:

| FOOD (SERVING) | BETA-CAROTENE (MG) |
| --- | --- |
| Spinach, cooked (½ cup) | 6.9 |
| Carrots, chopped, cooked (½ cup) | 6.5 |
| Collards, cooked (½ cup) | 5.8 |
| Carrots, raw (1 medium) | 5.1 |

| FOOD (SERVING) | BETA-CAROTENE (MG) |
|---|---|
| Cantaloupe, chopped (1 cup) | 3.2 |
| Sweet potato (1 whole) | 1.4 |
| Bell pepper, red, chopped, raw (½ cup) | 0.177 |

## RECIPE

# Golden Immunity Soup *Serves 2*

This recipe is packed with vitamin A. Make a large batch that you can meal prep and enjoy throughout the week! Serve this soup with some whole-grain bread.

¼ small yellow onion, peeled and diced

½ tablespoon extra-virgin olive oil

1 clove garlic, minced

¼ teaspoon ground turmeric

1 cup low-sodium vegetable broth

1 cup water

¼ cup lentils

1 medium stalk celery, chopped

¼ cup cubed sweet potato

1 medium carrot, peeled and chopped

½ medium zucchini, chopped

3 ounces canned diced tomatoes

¼ teaspoon dried oregano

¼ teaspoon crushed red pepper

⅛ teaspoon salt

⅛ teaspoon ground black pepper

¼ cup chopped kale

1 sprig fresh thyme

**PER SERVING**

*Calories: 181, Fat: 4g, Protein: 8g, Sodium: 345mg, Fiber: 6g, Carbohydrates: 31g, Sugar: 8g, Vitamin A: 8,193IU or 395mcg RAE*

1 In a large pot over medium heat, sauté onion in oil 3–5 minutes.

2 Add garlic and turmeric and cook another 1–2 minutes. Add broth and water and bring to a boil.

3 Add remaining ingredients, except for kale and thyme. Let simmer 40 minutes.

4 Add kale and thyme and cook 5 minutes or until kale is wilted.

5 Serve immediately.

# Amino Acids, Branched Chain
## (Isoleucine, Leucine, and Valine)

If you are into muscle building, you've probably heard of, or maybe even tried, branched-chain amino acids. Within the category of essential amino acids (AAs) are three special ones called branched-chain amino acids (BCAAs). The term "branched chain" refers to their chemical composition and the way they are linked together in a branching formation. These amino acids have important and specific roles both in normal body functions and in alleviating some serious medical conditions. Branched amino acids are a popular supplement, especially in the body-building community, but they are also in many foods that you are likely already eating. This entry will explore the pros and cons of these special amino acids.

### Description
Muscle protein synthesis occurs continuously in an attempt to replace the protein that is lost during protein breakdown. To synthesize new proteins, your body needs a sufficient amount of all essential amino acids—including branched-chain amino acids—as well as all nonessential amino acids. The BCAAs are used by the muscles, the heart, and the endocrine (hormone producing/regulating) system. The three BCAAs are:

- Isoleucine
- Leucine
- Valine

Some people take supplements that contain BCAAs hoping they will help pump up their muscles and boost their exercise performance and recovery. However, while BCAAs can increase muscle protein synthesis, they can't do so optimally without the other essential amino acids, such as those found in complete protein sources.

Some studies show that taking supplemental BCAAs helps with muscle building and reduces post-workout fatigue, while other studies show the opposite. The jury is still out on whether supplementing is ideal, but we do know that you should eat high-protein foods at most meals of the day. Doing so will help ensure you are meeting your needs because many foods containing protein (such as meat, fish, dairy, and tofu) also contain BCAAs.

In the hospital setting, BCAAs are given to patients who have liver disease, dyskinesia, and anorexia because it has been shown that they help with messaging mechanisms in the brain.

## Role in the Body
The different branched amino acids have different functions in the body:

### ISOLEUCINE:
- Involved in muscle metabolism
- Important for immune function
- Assists with hemoglobin production
- Is part of the body's energy regulation system

### LEUCINE:
- Helps regulate blood sugar levels
- Is critical for protein synthesis and muscle repair; also stimulates wound healing
- Produces growth hormones; leucine helps to activate a compound called mTOR, which helps cells to grow
- Helps with signaling between cells to ensure proper building of proteins

### VALINE:
- Works in partnership with the other BCAAs to build muscle tissue and other proteins in the body
- Helps with nitrogen balance in the body by working to eliminate extra nitrogen from the liver, preventing toxicity

- Is a "glucogenic amino acid," meaning it can be converted into glucose for energy

## Benefits
Following are some benefits of BCAAs:

- Build and maintain muscle
- Help reduce muscle soreness after a workout
- Leucine may decrease appetite, which can be helpful for weight management
- Provide an energy source in times of need
- Assist with proper cell signaling, especially during serious medical stress
- Help to preserve muscle mass

## Side Effects, Warnings, and Precautions
Consuming only BCAAs, or a disproportionate amount, without all the other essential amino acids may actually increase muscle protein breakdown. This is because *all* amino acids are needed for muscle protein synthesis. If only three essential amino acids are consumed, then protein breakdown is the only way the body can get the other amino acids required for synthesizing protein. Studies have shown a reduced muscle protein turnover during high BCAA intake. The turnover of protein is responsible for increased muscle efficiency. A reduction

will significantly decrease muscle strength in the long term.

Some studies also suggest that taking a high amount of BCAAs may induce insulin resistance by activation of mTOR. High doses of BCAA supplements can be harmful and can cause side effects such as nausea and headaches. They can also interfere with certain medicines, so make sure you talk with your doctor and dietitian if you take them as a supplement.

Overall, there is no strong evidence to support BCAA supplementation, especially in healthy individuals. Many trials have actually found negative effects of high BCAA intake. By getting all of your protein needs met by a variety of foods, you can ensure that proteins in your body are well balanced.

## Signs of Deficiency

Typically, only people with generalized protein deficiency are deficient in BCAA. If you are getting sufficient protein from food throughout the day, you are also getting enough BCAA. The signs of deficiency are the same as overall low protein, such as:

- Muscle wasting
- Weakness and fatigue
- Trouble concentrating

## How Much You Need

There are no official recommendations in the US for BCAA intake outside of the suggestions for overall protein intake. Recent studies indicate that BCAA needs may be as high as 67 milligrams per pound of body weight. An average daily intake of 15–30 grams of BCAA from the diet should meet most people's daily requirement. This amount can be easily obtained from food sources.

## Best Way to Consume

Getting BCAAs from complete protein sources is ideal, as they contain all the essential amino acids. Fortunately, BCAAs are abundantly found in many foods and whole-protein supplements. This makes BCAA supplements unnecessary for most people, especially if they consume enough protein in their diet. If you are unable to eat enough protein, or if you have certain medical issues, BCAA supplementation may be warranted and beneficial.

## Natural Food Sources

| FOOD (SERVING SIZE) | BCAA (G) | FOOD (SERVING SIZE) | BCAA (G) |
|---|---|---|---|
| Chicken (3 ounces) | 3 | Milk, any variety (1 cup) | 2 |
| Beef (3 ounces) | 3 | Tofu and tempeh (3 ounces) | 0.9–2.3 |
| Wild salmon (3 ounces) | 2.9 | Egg (1 large) | 1.3 |
| Beans and lentils, cooked (1 cup) | 2.5–3 | Quinoa (1 cup) | 1 |
| Cottage cheese (½ cup) | 2.3 | Nuts (1 ounce) | 0.7–1 |

## RECIPE

# Protein Booster Breakfast Skillet *Serves 1*

Get your protein boost first thing in the morning. This veggie-forward dish will leave you energized for a productive day.

½ tablespoon extra-virgin olive oil

¼ small onion, peeled and chopped

1 clove garlic, minced

½ small sweet potato, chopped

3 ounces tempeh, chopped

½ small red bell pepper, seeded and chopped

¼ cup black beans, rinsed and drained

1 large egg

Pinch salt

Pinch black pepper

1 tablespoon chopped fresh cilantro

4 cherry tomatoes, halved

**PER SERVING**
*Calories: 437, Fat: 19g, Protein: 28g, Sodium: 543mg, Fiber: 8g, Carbohydrates: 39g, Sugar: 7g*

1 Heat oil in a medium skillet over medium heat. Add onion and garlic. Cook 1–2 minutes.

2 Add potato, tempeh, bell pepper, and beans. Cook about 8–10 minutes or until potatoes are cooked through.

3 In the meantime, prepare egg in a small skillet to your liking.

4 When vegetables are cooked, add salt and pepper. Transfer to a serving bowl.

5 Serve egg over veggies, top with fresh cilantro and tomatoes, and enjoy!

# Amino Acids, Essential
## (Histidine, Isoleucine, Leucine, Lysine, Methionine, Phenylalanine, Threonine, Tryptophan, and Valine)

Amino acids (AA) are the building blocks of protein. Protein is one of the three essential macronutrients, along with carbohydrates and fat, that you need to consume daily. Your body can make some amino acids but others you have to get from the foods you eat. Out of twenty total amino acids in your body, there are nine that are essential. They are histidine, isoleucine, leucine, lysine, methionine, phenylalanine, threonine, tryptophan, and valine. Three of these essential AAs are called branched-chain amino acids (BCAAs) and are covered in the previous section, "Amino Acids, Branched Chain."

## Description

Amino acids are classified by whether or not they can be made by the body. Out of the twenty AAs that you use to make proteins, you need to get nine from the foods you eat; these are classified as "essential." Of the remaining eleven, five are considered "nonessential," meaning you can create them without having to eat them, and six are considered "conditionally essential," because you can only make them if you consume enough protein and other nutrients. In times of increased need, such as during severe illness, injury, or other stress to the body, you may need to consume these conditionally essential AAs like you would essential AAs.

In a nutshell:

- The nine essential amino acids are histidine, isoleucine, leucine, lysine, methionine, phenylalanine, threonine, tryptophan, and valine.
- The six conditionally essential amino acids are arginine (this AA is actually essential for children), cysteine, glutamine, glycine, proline, and tyrosine.
- The five nonessential amino acids are alanine, asparagine, aspartic acid, glutamic acid, and serine.

## Role in the Body

- **Muscle creation and maintenance:** Amino acids are the building blocks of proteins, which make up your muscles and tissues. Muscle cells turn over constantly and require protein to be remade and repaired. That's why it's important to also consume enough carbs and fats during meals so that protein can be used for muscle and tissue synthesis and repair.

- **Bone health:** Protein helps ensure proper bone development in kids and healthy bones throughout life. Sufficient protein intake in older adults can help to prevent bone fractures.
- **Weight loss and weight management:** Protein is necessary for your fullness mechanisms to work properly. It helps to reduce hunger and boost your metabolism. Some studies show that protein intakes consisting of 25–35 percent of your calories may help you lose weight and keep it off.
- **Repair and maintenance:** Amino acids are part of every single cell and tissue in the body, and a steady supply of them is needed for the constant rebuilding and repairing processes.
- **Creation of enzymes:** The compounds needed to speed up chemical reactions in the body—enzymes—are made of amino acids. Different combinations of amino acids create different enzymes. It takes one hundred to one thousand amino acids strung together to build an enzyme. Enzymes ensure that all kinds of chemical reactions, such as food digestion, happen efficiently.
- **Immune system health:** The ultimate protective barrier, your skin, is made from protein. Inside the body, other parts of the immune system such as antibodies and clotting factors are also made from amino acids.
- **Maintenance of healthy blood sugar levels:** Insulin, the messenger hormone that tells cells to take in sugar (glucose) from the blood, is made of fifty-one amino acids.
- **Help to form the key neurotransmitters:** Chemical messengers called neurotransmitters help transmit signals in the body. Three of these neurotransmitters—epinephrine, norepinephrine, and serotonin—affect mood and mental behavior. The essential AA tryptophan is needed for the synthesis of serotonin. Other AAs are also used by the brain to create various other neurotransmitters. The AAs act as precursors to the neurotransmitters, which means that they go through a series of chemical reactions and pairings with other compounds to ultimately produce neurotransmitters.
- **Energy source:** AAs form protein, which is not the body's preferred energy source, but in times of need, it can be used for energy.

## Benefits

- Promotes healthy muscle function
- Plays a role in weight loss and maintaining a weight
- Contributes to a healthy immune system and fewer illnesses

- In adequate amounts, assists in strengthening bones and reducing fracture risk
- Promotes healthy hair, skin, and nails
- Speeds up recovery from illness and injury
- Provides energy if other sources are insufficient
- May help lower blood pressure

## Side Effects, Warnings, and Precautions

If there are not sufficient carbohydrates and fats for energy, the body will begin to break down muscles for this purpose. That's why it's important to ensure that you are getting plenty of complex carbs and healthy fats, so that AAs can do all the essential functions that only they can do, instead of being used for energy.

While there's no upper limit for AA/protein amounts, people with kidney problems often need to avoid excess protein, as this can put a strain on the kidneys. Your doctor and dietitian should be consulted about how much protein you need if this is the case, as it will vary depending on the type of kidney condition.

## Signs of Deficiency

Mild protein deficiency (which is an overall low intake of all the various AAs) is actually quite common, and many people are at risk, in particular the elderly and people with illnesses. Athletes and those recovering from an injury or surgery require more protein as well. Being deficient in specific amino acids is not very common, but can occasionally happen with ones like tryptophan. This can impact some of the specific functions it has, like serotonin production. People who don't consume enough tryptophan may experience symptoms such as increased feelings of sadness and depression, since serotonin helps to regulate mood.

Globally, protein deficiency is a huge problem, affecting the growth and development of millions of children and the health of many adults. Kwashiorkor is a severe form of protein malnutrition that typically occurs in areas with insufficient food supply or famine. Children with kwashiorkor lose muscle mass and often have edema (accumulation of fluid beneath the skin due to the protein imbalance), weak immune systems, and anorexia.

Signs of deficiency can include:

- Increased appetite, which can, over time, lead to weight gain
- Loss of muscle mass
- Weakened immune system and increased susceptibility to infections
- Fatty liver
- Hair thinning and loss, weak nails, dry and flaky skin

- Weakened bones and increased fractures
- Edema (swelling of the skin due to fluid buildup)
- Stunting and delayed growth in children

## How Much You Need

The amount of protein (which includes all of the amino acids) you need depends on several factors, such as muscle mass, activity level, age, and weight, among others. There is no specific recommendation for AAs, since they are encompassed in the protein recommendations. Usually, protein needs are calculated based on body weight. The current Recommended Daily Allowance (RDA) for adults is 0.8 gram per kilogram, or 0.4 gram per pound of weight. This is likely enough for the *minimal* amount that most people need, but more recent research seems to indicate that this is below optimal. Following are general guidelines you can use to figure out some overall recommendations.

| AGE | MALE | FEMALE |
| --- | --- | --- |
| 0–6 months | 9g/day | 9g/day |
| 7–12 months | 11g/day | 11g/day |
| 1–3 years | 13g/day | 13g/day |
| 4–8 years | 19g/day | 19g/day |
| 9–13 years | 34g/day | 34g/day |

| AGE | MALE | FEMALE |
| --- | --- | --- |
| 14–18 years | 52g/day | 46g/day |
| 19–30 years | 56g/day | 46g/day |
| 31–50 years | 56g/day | 46g/day |
| 51+ years | 56g/day | 46g/day |
| Pregnancy | – | 71g/day |
| Lactation | – | 71g/day |

## Best Way to Consume

Almost all foods have some protein, and there are many excellent plant and animal sources. Many people would benefit from shifting to a more plant-based diet, and it's a good idea to try to eat plant sources of proteins for at least one third to one half of all meals. When you consume plant proteins, you're also getting all the other benefits that come with them, such as antioxidants, phytonutrients, vitamins, and minerals.

Fish is one of the top animal sources because it also contains healthy fats (omega-3s) and other valuable nutrients. There are other animal sources that tend to have more protein than most plant sources, but be cautious of excess red meat and fatty cuts of meat—the saturated fat in these cuts is the least-healthy type of fat and can lead to increased inflammation, a higher risk of heart disease, and other health problems.

## Natural Food Sources

Some animal-based food sources include:

| FOOD (SERVING SIZE) | PROTEIN (G) |
| --- | --- |
| Tuna (1 cup) | 39 |
| Cottage cheese, 2% fat (1 cup) | 27 |
| Chicken breast, roasted without skin (3 ounces) | 23 |
| Lean beef, cooked (3 ounces) | 22 |
| Greek yogurt, nonfat (6 ounces) | 17 |
| Egg (1 large) | 6 |

Some plant-based/vegan sources include:

| FOOD (SERVING SIZE) | PROTEIN (G) |
| --- | --- |
| Seitan (3½ ounces) | 25 |
| Tofu (3½ ounces) (protein content varies depending on soft versus firm) | 10–19 |
| Lentils, cooked (1 cup) | 18 |
| Quinoa, cooked (1 cup) | 8 |
| Almonds (2 tablespoons) | 6 |
| Hempseed (2 tablespoons) | 6 |
| Oats, raw (½ cup) | 6 |
| Hummus (¼ cup) | 5 |
| Broccoli, raw, chopped (1 cup) | 3 |

# Hummus Baked Chicken with Quinoa and Zucchini *Serves 1*

Hummus is delicious, is rich in protein, and provides a good source of iron. It also has a lot of heart-healthy fats. This recipe has 34 grams of protein and all of the essential amino acids.

½ cup chopped zucchini

½ medium green bell pepper, seeded and chopped

1 tablespoon extra-virgin olive oil

Pinch salt

Pinch black pepper

3 ounces boneless, skinless chicken breast, chopped into strips

4 tablespoons hummus

Juice of ½ medium lemon

¾ cup cooked quinoa

**PER SERVING**
*Calories: 506, Fat: 23g,*
*Protein: 32g, Sodium: 564mg,*
*Fiber: 9g, Carbohydrates: 44g,*
*Sugar: 5g*

1 Preheat oven to 450°F. Line a baking sheet with aluminum foil or spray with nonstick spray.

2 In a large bowl, combine zucchini and bell pepper with oil, salt, and pepper, then spread onto baking sheet.

3 Add chicken breast to the baking sheet and evenly coat with hummus.

4 Squeeze lemon juice over the chicken and veggies.

5 Bake 30–40 minutes or until chicken is cooked to an internal temperature of 165°F.

6 Serve chicken and vegetables immediately with quinoa, or let cool, cover, and store in the refrigerator.

# Peanut Noodles with Tofu *Serves 1*

Soba noodles are packed with protein and B vitamins. Combined with tofu and peanut butter, this Asian-inspired dish serves 30 grams of protein.

---

1 tablespoon extra-virgin olive oil

1 small red bell pepper, seeded and chopped

½ cup broccoli florets

4 ounces firm tofu, cubed

2 tablespoons peanut butter

2 tablespoons water

1 tablespoon plus 1½ teaspoons fresh lime juice, divided

2 teaspoons coconut aminos (or soy sauce)

1 teaspoon hot sauce

Pinch salt

Pinch black pepper

¾ cup soba (buckwheat) noodles, cooked

1 tablespoon chopped peanuts, for garnish

---

**PER SERVING**

*Calories: 576, Fat: 37g, Protein: 25g, Sodium: 631mg, Fiber: 6g, Carbohydrates: 40g, Sugar: 9g*

1 Heat oil in a medium skillet over medium heat. Add bell pepper and broccoli and sauté 5–6 minutes. Add tofu and cook 3 more minutes.

2 Add peanut butter, water, 1 tablespoon lime juice, coconut aminos, and hot sauce. Mix until the consistency is creamy. Add more water if desired. Add salt and pepper.

3 Add cooked noodles and stir to cover in peanut butter mixture. Transfer to a large serving bowl.

4 Serve with a sprinkling of crushed peanuts and a drizzle of remaining lime juice.

# Antioxidants

Possibly one of the buzziest terms in nutrition these days, it seems everyone wants more antioxidants. Like tiny warriors, antioxidants fight off and help stop cell and DNA damage due to oxidation, a destructive process that's constantly happening inside of your body. Antioxidants can help prevent cancer and heart disease, and can slow down aging, among other benefits. However, as usual, it is possible to have too much of a good thing, so getting the balance right—by getting your antioxidants from fresh, natural foods instead of taking pills—is extremely important.

## Description

"Antioxidant" is a general term that encompasses many different compounds. Antioxidants include vitamins, minerals, phytochemicals (plant complexes), plant pigments such as anthocyanins, and numerous others. Your body can produce some antioxidants, but to stay healthy, you need to get most of them from foods.

Antioxidants help to slow down or stop chemical chain reactions and processes like inflammation that ultimately lead to disease. Incredibly, they can help repair existing cell damage and undo some of the destruction caused by oxidation. Antioxidants also neutralize molecules called free radicals. Free radicals are essentially unstable atoms that are reactive and will damage your DNA and cells if not kept in check. Of note, recent research has shown that while free radicals do cause damage, they can also confer some benefits by stimulating cell regeneration, destroying harmful cells such as cancer cells, and striking back against bad bacteria in the body.

## Role in the Body

Each antioxidant has a special and unique role. For example, vitamin C's antioxidant prowess lies in its ability to scavenge free radicals from fluids inside and outside of your cells. Vitamin E, on the other hand, is fat-soluble, and helps to prevent oxidation in your fatty tissues. Scientific research shows that there are a plethora of other compounds that work synergistically with antioxidants to help them achieve their missions. These compounds come from whole-food sources, which is why it's so important to get antioxidants in this way. Many beneficial qualities are lost when the antioxidant is extracted to make a supplement or is created synthetically.

Here is a quick breakdown of some common antioxidants:

- **Vitamins:** Four of the thirteen vitamins act as antioxidants. They are vitamins $B_3$ (niacin), C, E, and beta-carotene (pro-vitamin A).
- **Minerals:** Four of the sixteen minerals act as antioxidants. They are selenium, zinc, copper, and manganese.
- **Plant compounds:** Plants produce compounds called phytonutrients to protect themselves from infections, bacteria, fungi, insects, and even the sun. Many, but not all, of these phytonutrients act as antioxidants. A few different categories of phytonutrients that have been studied include carotenoids, flavonoids (dark chocolate is a food rich in flavonoids—be sure to get 70 percent cocoa or higher to reap the benefits), organosulfur compounds (foods like onions, leeks, and garlic), and phenolic phytonutrients from herbs and spices.

## Benefits

There are numerous benefits to antioxidants, including:

- **Fighting aging:** Antioxidants protect your cells from oxidative damage that accelerates the aging process. Recent research on telomeres, which are DNA sequences found at the ends of your chromosomes that get shorter as you grow older, indicates that antioxidants can help maintain telomere length.

- **Preventing chronic disease:** Oxidation of lipids and protein produces free radicals in the body, which can increase the risk of chronic diseases such as heart disease, cancer, and cataracts. Antioxidants can safely pick up some of the toxins produced from oxidation in the body and remove or neutralize them.

- **Supporting immune functions:** Natural antioxidants help defend the body against toxins and harmful materials that might cause inflammatory responses, infections, and cell damage. Antioxidants also help fight against viral and bacterial infections, as well as reduce inflammation caused by autoimmune diseases like rheumatoid arthritis.

## Side Effects, Warnings, and Precautions

High doses of antioxidants can have the reverse effect of what is desired. Instead of reducing oxidation, too high a dose of antioxidants can promote it. Some free radicals are actually protective, and taking too many antioxidants—which would only be possible by taking supplements—can destroy or slow down protective free radicals.

Antioxidant supplements, like vitamins C and E, can decrease the efficacy of some cancer treatments. Always discuss everything you are taking with your doctor and dietitian if you are receiving medical treatment.

## Signs of Deficiency
Signs of deficiency can include:

- Fatigue, lack of energy
- Changes in skin and hair—increased aging and brittle hair
- Poor memory and "brain fog"
- Acceleration of diet-related chronic diseases such as heart disease, diabetes, and cancer

## How Much You Need
There is no established Recommended Daily Allowance (RDA) for antioxidants, but a good way to ensure you are getting enough is to meet the daily recommended intake for fruits and vegetables. The recommended amount for adults is 1½–2 cups per day of fruit and 2–3 cups per day of vegetables. For children, 1–1½ cups per day of fruit and 1–2 cups per day of vegetables is sufficient.

## Best Way to Consume
Antioxidants are mostly found in plant foods. Make sure your diet is full of colorful fruits and vegetables, as a variety of colors signifies different types of antioxidants. This is one reason why it's important to "eat the rainbow."

Antioxidant content begins to decline as soon as the fruit or vegetable is picked or harvested. Ideally, you should be selecting fruits and vegetables that are grown as close to you as possible. Try visiting a local farmers' market, planting your own garden, or, if you have limited space, placing a potted herb plant on your counter.

## Natural Food Sources
Here are some foods that contain the most antioxidants:

### BERRIES
- Amla berry: Indian gooseberry; ranks extremely high in antioxidant quantity
- Bilberry
- Blackberry
- Blueberry
- Chokeberry: native to eastern North America
- Barberry: known as *zereshk*; commonly used in Iranian cuisine
- Dog rose berry: usually used to make tea; native to Europe, Africa, and Asia
- Sour cherry
- Raspberry
- Red whortleberry: known as lingonberry; common to Norway

### FRUITS
- Apricots
- Grapes, blue
- Pomegranates
- Olives, black, Kalamata
- Plums

- Prunes
- Mangoes

**HERBS AND MEDICINAL PLANTS**
- Arjuna, powder in capsule: native to India
- Arnica, flower and seeds, dried: originated in Germany
- Cascara sagrada: originated in Mexico
- *Cinnamomi cortex*: used in traditional Korean medicine
- *Sangre de Grado*, liquid solution: from the Amazon region of South America
- Triphala, powder in capsule: native to India

**LEGUMES**
- Lentils, green
- Pinto beans
- Soyatein (protein-rich soya)
- Soybeans, white, small size, dry
- Navy beans, dry

**NUTS**
- Chestnuts
- Flaxseed, ground
- Kernel from watermelon, roasted with salt and spices (commonly consumed in Iran)
- Peanuts, roasted
- Pecans
- Pistachios
- Walnuts
- Sunflower seeds

**SPICES**
- Allspice, dried, ground: commonly used in southern Mexico and Central America
- Alpine lady's mantle, leaves, dried: widespread in Britain and Ireland
- Barberry, bark: native to Europe and Iran
- Bearberry, leaves, dried: used as tea
- Blackcurrant, leaves, dried: oil, leaves, fruits, and flower can be used as medicine; native to central and northern Europe and northern Asia
- Cinnamon, dried ground
- Clove, dried ground: native to Indonesia, used in the cuisines of Asia, Africa, and the Middle East
- Coltsfoot, leaves, dried: native to northern Europe and Asia
- Common butterwort, leaves, dried: originated in Europe and North America; used as herbal tea
- Dill, dried
- Green mint, leaves, dried
- Juniper berries, green, dried: mostly grown in North Africa; normally used as tea
- Lemon balm, leaves: dried leaves used as tea and ointments; fresh leaves used as essential oils
- Lemon thyme, leaves and flower, dried

**VEGETABLES**

- Curly kale
- Leaves from the African baobab tree, dry, crushed: consumed in parts of Africa
- Bell peppers
- Spinach
- Artichokes
- Broccoli
- Cabbage
- Tomato juice

**RECIPE**

# Dark Chocolate Mousse with Blueberries and Strawberries

*Serves 2*

Would you believe there is a dessert that is good for you? If your answer is no, this one will change your mind. Packed with antioxidants and healthy fats, it makes for a perfect dessert or even a sweet snack!

| | | |
|---|---|---|
| 1 medium ripe avocado, peeled, pitted, and sliced | 1 tablespoon creamy almond butter | 2 tablespoons unsweetened cocoa powder |
| 1 medium ripe banana, peeled and sliced | 1 tablespoon agave | 4 medium strawberries |
| ¼ cup almond milk | | ¼ cup blueberries |

**PER SERVING**

*Calories: 269, Fat: 14g, Protein: 5g, Sodium: 25mg, Fiber: 10g, Carbohydrates: 34g, Sugar: 16g*

1 In a blender or food processor, combine all ingredients except the berries and mix until smooth.
2 Chill in the refrigerator 30 minutes to 2 hours.
3 Garnish with strawberries and blueberries and serve.

# Vitamin B₁: Thiamin

Even though thiamin doesn't get as much attention as some of the other vitamins, its role in the body is remarkable. This vitamin is essential for normal growth and development, helps regulate your metabolism, and is needed for energy production in most cells inside of your body. There are some conditions that may require supplementation, which will be described further in this section, but for the majority of people, eating a balanced diet will provide enough thiamin for optimal health.

## Description

Vitamin $B_1$, also called thiamin, was the first B-complex vitamin to be discovered. Similar to all other B vitamins, thiamin is water-soluble. Water-soluble vitamins are not stored in the body, and so regular intake is required. A small amount of thiamin is stored in the liver, but because thiamin has a short half-life (the amount of time it takes for half of it to degrade and no longer be usable) of about two weeks, consistent intake is important.

Since most Americans consume fortified grain products regularly, deficiency is now rare in the US. However, before fortification began in the 1940s, thiamin deficiency was quite common,

sometimes leading to a serious condition called beriberi (see "Signs of Deficiency").

## Role in the Body

Recent research studies have documented a relationship between Alzheimer's disease development and thiamin deficiency. It seems that getting the right amount of thiamin prior to middle age may be important to preventing dementia as we grow older. This makes sense because thiamin is important to proper brain functioning and conversion of nutrients into energy in the brain.

Here are more of thiamin's functions.

- Thiamin is necessary for the production of cellular energy—and it is especially related to proper heart, nervous system, and gastrointestinal (GI) system functioning.
- Thiamin helps the body convert carbohydrates and fats into energy.
- It acts as a coenzyme for many important reactions in the body such as converting blood sugar into energy in your brain, key processes in your heart tissues, forming red blood cells, and converting nutrients from the foods you eat into forms that your cells can use.

## Benefits

- It is required for the conversion of tryptophan (an amino acid) into serotonin, a neurotransmitter that helps to regulate mood, anxiety, and body temperature. Serotonin also plays a role in learning and memory.
- It helps the transport of electrolytes in and out of your cells, ensuring that your heart and muscles can contract and function well.
- Sufficient levels of thiamin keep your organs and systems working properly. It's key for brain function and nervous system optimization.
- It is important for digestive function.
- It may be helpful for diabetics by improving circulation and blood flow.

## Side Effects, Warnings, and Precautions

Dietary consumption of thiamin is extremely safe and the only known interactions are from supplements. There are no known serious interactions between thiamin and medications, but a small number of people may develop an allergic reaction to high-dose supplements of B vitamins. However, moderate interactions of thiamin (such as itching or hives) can occur with specific oral antibiotics such as azithromycin and clarithromycin.

Pregnant women are advised not to exceed the recommended amount of thiamin, as the impact of a high thiamin intake level on a baby's development has not yet been determined.

In terms of other interactions, chewing betel nuts (areca)—as is popular in many countries in Asia and East Africa—interferes with thiamin absorption.

## Signs of Deficiency

Overall, the most common signs of a severe thiamin deficiency are neurological symptoms such as walking unsteadily, memory loss, and muscle weakness. Since thiamin is so important in energy conversion and brain functioning, a severe deficiency impairs proper functioning of the brain and nervous system, heart, muscles, and GI system. The two most common thiamin-deficiency disorders are beriberi (characterized by muscle atrophy and numbness in the fingers and toes) and a neurological disorder called Wernicke–Korsakoff syndrome (most commonly related to malnutrition and alcoholism).

In the US, thiamin deficiency is not common, except among the following:

- **People with alcohol dependence:** Chronic alcohol abuse leads to reduced thiamin absorption in the gut and interferes with thiamin storage in the liver, as well as thiamin phosphorylation (activation so it can do its job properly).

- **The elderly:** As many as 30 percent of older adults may be low in thiamin. The causes include reduced consumption of thiamin-containing foods, medications that interact with thiamin absorption, chronic disease, and reduced absorption as part of aging.
- **Individuals with HIV/AIDS:** Some research suggests that low thiamin is underdiagnosed in those with HIV/AIDS, but more data is needed.
- **Diabetics:** Research has indicated that type 1 diabetics have much lower (around 75 percent) levels of thiamin than average, and type 2 diabetics could have 50–75 percent lower thiamin. It could be due to enzymatic activity or increased clearance by the kidneys.
- **Bariatric surgery patients:** One of the risks of weight loss surgery is severe thiamin deficiency because absorption of nutrients is drastically decreased.

## How Much You Need (RDA)

| AGE | MALE | FEMALE |
| --- | --- | --- |
| 0–6 months | 0.2mg | 0.2mg |
| 7–12 months | 0.3mg | 0.3mg |
| 1–3 years | 0.5mg | 0.5mg |
| 4–8 years | 0.6mg | 0.6mg |
| 9–13 years | 0.9mg | 0.9mg |
| 14–18 years | 1.2mg | 1.0mg |

| AGE | MALE | FEMALE |
| --- | --- | --- |
| 19–50 years | 1.2mcg | 1.1mcg |
| 51+ years | 1.2mcg | 1.1mcg |
| Pregnancy | – | 1.4mcg |
| Lactation | – | 1.4mcg |

There is no upper limit for thiamin, because any excess is excreted in urine. Even at very high intakes (50 milligrams/day or higher), no negative effects have been reported.

## Best Way to Consume

You can find thiamin in a wide range of foods, including seafood, beef, pork, legumes, whole grains, and acorn squash. It's also included in many fortified products such as pasta and bread. Eating whole-grain products within a balanced daily diet is the best way to consume enough thiamin, but a daily intake of all B-complex vitamins is necessary for thiamin to be effectively absorbed into the blood. Whole grains are higher in thiamin than their processed counterparts.

Poor absorption of thiamin in the gut has been linked to the use of diuretics, gastric bypass surgery, and GI conditions, such as gluten sensitivity, adversely impacting nutrient absorption.

## Natural Food Sources

| FOOD (SERVING SIZE) | THIAMIN (MG) |
| --- | --- |
| Breakfast cereals (fortified with 100% of the Daily Value for thiamin) (1 serving) | 1.5 |
| Egg noodles, enriched, cooked (1 cup) | 0.5 |
| Pork chop, cooked (3 ounces) | 0.4 |
| Fresh trout, cooked (3 ounces) | 0.4 |
| Fresh tuna, cooked (3 ounces) | 0.2 |
| Brown rice, natural, long grain, cooked (½ cup) | 0.1 |
| Yogurt, plain, low-fat (1 cup) | 0.1 |
| Sunflower seeds, toasted (1 ounce) | 0.1 |

## RECIPE

# Peanut Butter Cup Overnight Oats *Serves 3*

This easy and delicious breakfast is not only a great source of thiamin; it is also full of fiber, healthy fats, and antioxidants. Feel free to substitute the maple syrup with honey if you prefer and choose another nut butter if peanut butter isn't your thing.

1½ cups rolled oats

3 tablespoons unsweetened cocoa powder

1½ cups low-fat milk (or any kind you prefer)

1½ teaspoons vanilla extract

2 tablespoons pure maple syrup

2 tablespoons peanut butter

1 tablespoon dark chocolate chips

**PER SERVING**

*Calories: 257, Fat: 8g, Protein: 12g, Sodium: 59mg, Fiber: 7g, Carbohydrates: 42g, Sugar: 2g, Thiamin: 0.31mg*

1 In an 8-ounce Mason jar or small, sealable container, combine all ingredients. Stir.

2 Cover with a lid or plastic wrap and refrigerate at least 8 hours (overnight is best).

3 Serve.

# Vitamin B$_2$: Riboflavin

Riboflavin, also known as vitamin B$_2$, is a bright yellow nutritional superstar. Its name comes from the Latin word for "yellow": *flavus*. The second of the B-complex vitamins, riboflavin is needed for energy production, allows oxygen to be properly used by the body, and has a plethora of other important functions. Riboflavin can be destroyed by sunlight, which is the reason why milk is now mainly sold in opaque cartons rather than glass containers.

## Description
Getting enough riboflavin from your diet isn't too difficult. Many foods are fortified with this essential nutrient, and some animal products are also a rich source of it. There are a few vegetarian sources as well, and you might be surprised to learn that bacteria in your large intestine can produce small amounts of riboflavin. Interestingly, that same bacteria can produce a bit more of the vitamin after you eat vegetable-based rather than meat-based foods.

Aside from the critical role that vitamin B$_2$ plays in activating energy pathways, it's important for your body's detox system. Some research studies have shown that it may also help with issues such as migraine headaches.

## Role in the Body
Riboflavin from the foods you eat is mainly absorbed in the small intestine. It's optimal to get a steady daily amount because it's only absorbed in small doses. Anything else is flushed out quickly. Here are some of riboflavin's functions:

- Riboflavin helps activate pathways that are integral to the production of energy, growth, development, and daily activities. These pathways also play a role in the metabolism (and, thus, detoxification) of fats and drugs.
- Riboflavin keeps levels of certain nutrients in the right balance. For example, the nutrient homocysteine (which is a type of amino acid) is important but also needs to be kept in check, because high levels of it are linked to heart disease. You mostly get homocysteine from eating meat, but riboflavin plus other B vitamins help to maintain normal levels of it in the blood. If you don't consume enough riboflavin, it could cause elevated homocysteine and raise your risk for heart disease.

## Benefits
Vitamin B$_2$ can be beneficial for people who suffer from migraines. Taking extra

B$_2$ has been shown to be an excellent preventive measure by some research studies. Taking 200 milligrams per day may help to alleviate migraine symptoms in some people. Additionally, athletes tend to require extra riboflavin to help replenish all the energy they are using up.

## Side Effects, Warnings, and Precautions

Too much vitamin B$_2$ is rare, especially if you're getting your vitamins from food—which is almost always the ideal! However, super high doses from B$_2$ vitamins can cause side effects such as rash, diarrhea, or increased urination.

## Signs of Deficiency

Low vitamin B$_2$ is very rare in developed nations. People with a poor diet, the elderly, and people who abuse alcohol tend to be most at risk for low riboflavin. Also, lung disease seems to increase the risk of deficiency. Very low levels of B$_2$ will result in symptoms that include skin and eye problems, a sore throat, a swollen tongue, and anemia. This condition is called ariboflavinosis and is rare. Since B$_2$ works in synergy with other B vitamins and some of the protein building blocks, extremely low levels of it will cause low levels or improper conversions of B$_6$ and niacin.

## How Much You Need (RDA)

| AGE | MALE | FEMALE |
| --- | --- | --- |
| 0–6 months | 0.3mg (AI not RDA)* | 0.3mg (AI not RDA)* |
| 7–12 months | 0.4mg (AI not RDA)* | 0.4mg (AI not RDA)* |
| 1–3 years | 0.5mg | 0.5mg |
| 4–8 years | 0.6mg | 0.6mg |
| 9–13 years | 0.9mg | 0.9mg |
| 14–18 years | 1.3mg | 1.0mg |
| 19–50 years | 1.3mg | 1.1mg |
| 51+ years | 1.3mg | 1.1mg |
| Pregnancy | – | 1.4mg |
| Lactation | – | 1.6mg |

* Adequate Intake amounts were developed for infants because there isn't sufficient evidence for a Recommended Daily Allowance (RDA).

There is no upper limit for riboflavin, because any excess is quickly excreted. No negative effects have been reported even at high intakes. Your body carefully controls how much is absorbed, so once the limit is reached, the rest is eliminated.

## Best Way to Consume

This vitamin, part of the water-soluble B group, is available in multiple forms. It occurs naturally in many foods, including eggs, green vegetables, meat, and almonds. It is also often added through fortification to milled foods, where the milling process has removed it.

## Natural Food Sources

| FOOD (SERVING SIZE) | RIBOFLAVIN (MG) |
| --- | --- |
| Beef liver, pan fried (3 ounces) | 2.9 |
| Oats, instant, fortified, cooked with water (1 cup) | 1.1 |
| Yogurt, plain, fat-free (1 cup) | 0.6 |
| Milk, 2% fat (1 cup) | 0.5 |
| Clams, cooked, moist heat (3 ounces) | 0.4 |
| Mushrooms, portabella, sliced,grilled (½ cup) | 0.3 |
| Almonds, dry roasted (1 ounce) | 0.3 |
| Crab, cooked (3½ ounces) | 0.2 |
| Quinoa, cooked (1 cup) | 0.2 |

## RECIPE

# Avocado and Crab Salad  *Serves 2*

This super creamy salad is rich in $B_2$, healthy fats, and protein. It's bursting with zest and flavor. For optimal freshness, eat this salad the day of or the day after preparation.

1 (6-ounce) can crab meat, drained and flaked

1 large hard-boiled egg, sliced

1 cup baby spinach

½ medium avocado, peeled, pitted, and mashed

1 small yellow bell pepper, seeded and chopped

¼ small onion, peeled and diced

1 tablespoon sunflower seeds

½ tablespoon minced garlic

½ teaspoon cayenne pepper

Juice from ½ medium lime

2 tablespoons chopped fresh cilantro

2 slices whole-grain bread, toasted

**PER SERVING**

*Calories: 296, Fat: 11g, Protein: 25g, Sodium: 624mg, Fiber: 6g, Carbohydrates: 24g, Sugar: 3g, Riboflavin: 0.35mg*

1  In a medium bowl, combine crab, egg, spinach, avocado, bell pepper, onion, sunflower seeds, garlic, cayenne pepper, and lime juice. Top with cilantro.

2  Serve with toasted bread.

# Vitamin $B_3$: Niacin

Niacin was discovered in 1937 through the diligent experiments of American biochemist Conrad Arnold Elvehjem and the work of Austrian-American doctor Joseph Goldberger, as well Dr. Tom Spies. These scientists discovered that deficiency could be induced by limiting certain foods—they just had to figure out which ones. Elvehjem induced niacin deficiency in dogs, which turned their tongues black, then reversed it by feeding them foods rich in niacin. Dr. Spies helped to confirm those findings. After this discovery, the debilitating effects of niacin deficiency (known in its most severe form as pellagra), which affected millions of people, were massively reduced—a huge public health success.

## Description

This essential vitamin is found naturally in a broad range of foods, but especially in fish, poultry, beef, nuts, legumes, yeast, and some grains. (It is also found in many fortified food items, such as breakfast cereals.) Additionally, niacin can be made in the body from tryptophan, an essential amino acid. For niacin to be produced in the body from tryptophan, sufficient amounts of the following vitamins and minerals must also be in the blood: vitamin $B_2$ (riboflavin), vitamin $B_6$ (pyridoxine), iron, and copper.

The main function of niacin is to convert food—carbohydrates, fats, and protein—into energy and enzymes. Niacin gets converted into the coenzymes nicotinamide adenine dinucleotide (NAD) and nicotinamide adenine dinucleotide phosphate (NADP) inside most tissues in the body. The amazing thing about NAD is that it helps over 400 different enzymes to activate various processes in the body—that's more than any other vitamin!

## Role in the Body

- Niacin's primary role is the creation of energy at the cellular level (which produces energy at the level of the tissues and organs).
- NAD and NADP also interact closely with adenosine triphosphate (ATP), an essential component of cellular respiration, which results in energy that enables the body's organs to function.
- Niacin plays a role in enabling proper gland and liver function.
- Niacin has been linked to lowering the blood level of LDL (the "bad" cholesterol).

## Benefits

Since dementia can be caused by niacin deficiency—and niacin deficiency is associated with premature aging—various studies are currently investigating whether niacin supplements can slow the progression of Parkinson's disease and Alzheimer's disease. The authors of a 2004 research article in *The Journal of Neurology, Neurosurgery, and Psychiatry* concluded that niacin supplementation in people with niacin deficiencies could slow Alzheimer's disease progression. A 2018 article in *The International Journal of Tryptophan Research* suggested that niacin plays a protective role against Parkinson's disease.

Niacin also:

- Helps to provide energy for the brain to function (the feeling of "brain fog" can be caused by niacin deficiency)
- Decreases risk of cardiovascular disease
- May be protective against diabetes

## Side Effects, Warnings, and Precautions

Getting too much (which would only be possible by taking supplements) niacin can cause adverse side effects. These include flushing, dizziness, rapid heartbeat, and liver damage.

According to research, 20 percent of people who take niacin supplements in daily doses of 500 milligrams or higher develop elevated levels of serum aminotransferase, an indicator of liver toxicity.

Niacin can interact with certain medications, such as isoniazid (used to treat tuberculosis) and anti-diabetes medications. People with diabetes taking nicotinic (a form of niacin) acid supplements should have their glucose levels carefully monitored, since these supplements are linked to increased glucose levels.

## Signs of Deficiency

Niacin deficiency is common in impoverished global regions, due to a high daily consumption of only unfortified grains such as cornmeal. In developed countries deficiency is frequently associated with alcoholism or bacterial overgrowth in the intestinal tract (which interferes with nutrient absorption).

The vitamin-deficiency disorder most associated with a severe niacin deficiency is pellagra. The primary symptoms of this potentially fatal disorder are known as the four Ds—dermatitis, diarrhea, dementia, and death—and it was first linked to a severe niacin deficiency in 1937. Pellagra is considered an extremely serious disorder requiring immediate medical attention.

Dry, cracked skin is common in niacin-deficient people. Another related symptom is inflammation of the mucus membranes (and inflammation of the intestinal tract is also common).

## How Much You Need

The following is the RDA for niacin:

| AGE | MALE | FEMALE |
|---|---|---|
| 0–6 months | 2mg (AI not RDA)* | 2mg (AI not RDA)* |
| 7–12 months | 4mg (AI not RDA)* | 4mg (AI not RDA)* |
| 1–3 years | 6mg | 6mg |
| 4–8 years | 8mg | 8mg |
| 9–13 years | 12mg | 12mg |
| 14–18 years | 16mg | 14mg |
| 19+ years | 16mg | 14mg |
| Pregnancy | – | 18mg |
| Lactation | – | 17mg |

* Adequate Intake amounts were developed for infants because there isn't sufficient evidence for a Recommended Daily Allowance (RDA).

## Best Way to Consume

Eating daily balanced meals is the best way to consume niacin. While grains are a source, poultry, fish, nuts, and legumes contain more niacin. However your daily niacin is obtained, it is important to recognize that sufficient quantities of all B-complex vitamins are necessary for niacin to be adequately absorbed. People with anorexia or bulimia are classified in an "under-nutritional status" and are at higher risk of niacin deficiency.

In addition, people with an inadequate intake of riboflavin, pyridoxine, and/or iron may experience a niacin deficiency, since a lack of these three nutrients impedes the conversion of tryptophan to niacin. This is because the coenzymes in the metabolic pathway depend on these three nutrients to function properly.

## Natural Food Sources

| FOOD (SERVING SIZE) | NIACIN (MG) |
|---|---|
| Beef liver, pan fried (3 ounces) | 14.9 |
| Chicken breast, meat only, grilled (3 ounces) | 10.3 |
| Marinara sauce, ready to serve (1 cup) | 10.3 |
| Turkey breast, meat only, roasted (3 ounces) | 10.0 |
| Salmon, sockeye, cooked (3 ounces) | 8.6 |
| Tuna, light, canned in water, drained (3 ounces) | 8.6 |
| Peanuts, dry roasted (1 ounce) | 4.2 |
| Rice, white, enriched, cooked (1 cup) | 2.3 |

# Kale Salad with Chicken *Serves 1*

This niacin-rich recipe is a perfect lunch for busier days. Pack it up and enjoy a healthy break between meetings! It's easy to prepare the night before and you can save even more time by getting precooked chicken to add to the rest of the salad.

---

### SALAD

1 small boneless, skinless chicken breast (about 4 ounces)

1 cup chopped kale

1 small tomato, chopped

½ cup halved strawberries

⅓ medium red onion, peeled and sliced

1 tablespoon chopped walnuts

### DRESSING

¼ cup balsamic vinegar

1 tablespoon olive oil

1 tablespoon Dijon mustard

1 tablespoon honey

1/16 teaspoon salt

⅛ teaspoon black pepper

---

**PER SERVING**
*Calories: 503, Fat: 22g, Protein: 32g, Sodium: 589mg, Fiber: 4g, Carbohydrates: 44g, Sugar: 34g, Niacin: 11.8mg*

1 Preheat oven to 400°F. Spray a baking sheet with nonstick cooking spray.

2 Place chicken on baking sheet and cook 25–40 minutes or until internal temperature reads 165°F. Set aside to let cool.

3 In a medium bowl, toss together kale, tomato, strawberries, onion, and walnuts.

4 Cut chicken into strips and add to other ingredients.

5 In a small bowl, mix all dressing ingredients together. Add as much as desired to salad just before eating and toss to coat. Store any remaining dressing in the fridge.

# Vitamin B₅: Pantothenic Acid

Vitamin $B_5$ (also called pantothenic acid) is essential to help create bursts of energy that enable your organs and muscles to function and fire properly. Fortunately, vitamin $B_5$ is contained in most animal-based and plant-based foods. Vitamin $B_5$ is also added to many food products (such as most breakfast cereals). This means that a *solely* diet-related vitamin $B_5$ deficiency is rare except among people with severe mal-nutrition (it does occur in rural Africa and other impoverished areas that experience seasonal food scarcity). Like its other B vitamin family members, $B_5$ is water-soluble, so it's excreted in urine. For this reason, you need to have a daily intake of $B_5$ to stay healthy—but you'll see that's easy to do because it's found in such a wide variety of foods!

## Description

Unlike many other B vitamins, vitamin $B_5$ primarily functions by enabling enzymes to act properly, thereby allowing essential processes in your body to occur at a biochemical level. In particular, vitamin $B_5$ plays a role in the production of coenzyme A (coA), which is involved in the synthesis and oxidation of fatty acids. In turn, fatty acids are necessary for the formation of fats. And fats are an alternate energy source for your body after its main energy source, carbohydrates. It is important to note that cooking foods containing vitamin $B_5$ can destroy up to 80 percent of the vitamin.

## Role in the Body

- Vitamin $B_5$ functions at the cellular level in the body so your tissues and organ systems can run smoothly.
- It is necessary for red blood cell creation, synthesizing of cholesterol, and the creation of stress hormones (like adrenaline) and reproductive hormones.
- It is needed for the creation of the brain neurotransmitter acetylcholine, which causes muscles to contract.
- This vitamin is necessary in an adequate amount for the proper absorption of the other B vitamins. In this way, vitamin $B_5$ affects an even wider range of biochemical processes than simply those specifically associated with it.

## Benefits

Besides the benefit of enabling—from a cellular perspective—the energy necessary for life, there are a wide range of other benefits associated with adequate vitamin B5 daily intake.

- Study findings have suggested a link between pantothenic acid supplementation and decreased production of LDL ("bad" cholesterol).
- Other researchers have suggested that vitamin B5 contributes to moisturizing skin. Their conclusions about potential skin benefits are based on in vitro studies performed in scientific laboratories showing that pantothenic acid is essential for the generation of keratinocytes—and keratinocytes are fundamental for healthy skin.
- There are claims that pantothenic acid can treat nerve damage, improve mental ability, prevent arthritis, and prevent diverse birth defects, but these findings have not been substantiated by current scientific evidence.

## Side Effects, Warnings, and Precautions

Since vitamin B5 is excreted each day in the urine, no maximum daily recommended intake has been established. However, ingesting too high a dose of pantothenic acid may induce diarrhea in some people. There are no specific warnings linked to the ingestion of vitamin B5, except that people should cease taking a pantothenic acid supplement if an allergic reaction to it occurs.

## Signs of Deficiency

Vitamin B5 deficiency has only been documented among people with malnutrition. Since this condition can occur in people suffering from moderate to severe anorexia or long-standing alcoholism, people diagnosed with either are at far higher risk for vitamin B5 deficiency than those outside these groups.

The common signs of deficiency include:

- Generalized malaise and/or tiredness
- Numbness and tingling in the lower extremities

Pantothenate kinase–associated neurodegeneration (PKAN) (formerly called Hallervorden-Spatz syndrome), is a hereditary disorder linked to a pantothenic acid metabolism gene abnormality. This congenital disorder is characterized by progressive degeneration of specific regions in the central nervous system (CNS). Only one to three babies in every three million births are born with PKAN.

## How Much You Need

There currently is no agreed-upon RDA for vitamin B5. This lack of consensus is due to the fact that deficiencies have only been found in people suffering from severe malnutrition. Instead, a daily Adequate Intake (AI) has been given:

Intake at this level is assumed to ensure nutritional adequacy; it is established when evidence is insufficient to develop an RDA. Adequate Intake for vitamin $B_5$ is as follows:

| AGE | MALE | FEMALE |
| --- | --- | --- |
| 0–12 months | 1.7–1.8mg | 1.7–1.8mg |
| 1–3 years | 2mg | 2mg |
| 4–8 years | 3mg | 3mg |
| 9–13 years | 4mg | 4mg |
| 14–18 years | 5mg | 5mg |
| 19+ years | 5mg | 5mg |
| Pregnancy | – | 6mg |
| Lactation | – | 7mg |

## Best Way to Consume

The best way to absorb vitamin $B_5$ is by eating foods that contain it. The following are particularly excellent sources of vitamin $B_5$:

- Dried brewer's yeast
- Beef and chicken liver
- Peanut butter
- Soybeans

For people with intestinal disorders (such as Crohn's disease) that interfere with the absorption of nutrients from food, boosting the level of vitamin $B_5$ by taking a pantothenic acid supplement may be necessary.

## Natural Food Sources

| FOOD (SERVING SIZE) | PANTOTHENIC ACID (MG) |
| --- | --- |
| Yogurt, low-fat, plain (8 ounces) | 1.3 |
| Sunflower seeds (¼ cup) | 2.4 |
| Egg, hard-boiled (1 large) | 0.7 |
| Broccoli, chopped, boiled, drained (½ cup) | 0.5 |
| Rice, brown, medium-grain, cooked (½ cup) | 0.4 |
| Cheddar cheese (1½ ounces) | 0.2 |

Additional sources of vitamin B pantothenic acid include fortified foods. It is useful to read the packaging label to determine if—and how much—pantothenic acid has been added to the product.

# Loaded Avocado Toast *Serves 1*

If you want to spice up this dish, add some hot sauce on top.

---

1 teaspoon extra-virgin olive oil

½ cup sliced mushrooms

1 slice whole-wheat bread, toasted

½ medium avocado, peeled, pitted, and mashed

1 large hard-boiled egg, sliced

1 tablespoon sunflower seeds

¼ cup broccoli sprouts

Pinch salt

Pinch black pepper

---

**PER SERVING**

*Calories: 368, Fat: 24g, Protein: 14g, Sodium: 503mg, Fiber: 8g, Carbohydrates: 23g, Sugar: 3g, Pantothenic Acid: 3.1mg*

1 Heat oil in a medium pan over medium heat. Add mushrooms and cook until soft, about 3–5 minutes. Set aside.

2 Place toasted bread on a work surface and add mashed avocado, cooked mushrooms, egg, sunflower seeds, and sprouts.

3 Season with salt and pepper and serve.

# Vitamin $B_6$

Vitamin $B_6$ is a water-soluble vitamin naturally found in a wide variety of foods. It can also be added back into foods where it was lost during processing (known as enrichment) or consumed as a dietary supplement. Vitamin $B_6$ deficiency is rare in developed countries. However, alcoholics, women taking contraceptive pills, and people with thyroid, autoimmune, and renal problems can be at risk of deficiency. Vitamin $B_6$ deficiency is usually associated with deficiencies of other B vitamins, such as folic acid and vitamin $B_{12}$. Although $B_6$ is not as "famous" as some of the other Bs, it plays an important role in maintaining important bodily functions and is essential for good health.

## Description

Vitamin $B_6$ is actually not a single vitamin but a group of six different compounds that include pyridoxamine, pyridoxine, pyridoxal, and other phosphorylated forms. It's found in many different foods, but how well it is absorbed from the foods varies, depending on the form it is found in. For example, some of the naturally occurring $B_6$ in many plant foods is not as well absorbed from them as from animal foods because it comes in a form that's not as bioavailable.

## Role in the Body

- Vitamin $B_6$ is a coenzyme involved in more than 140 biochemical reactions in the cells, including protein, carbohydrate, and lipid metabolism; hemoglobin formation; neurotransmitter synthesis; and production of IL-2 by lymphocytes.
- Studies have shown that vitamin $B_6$ can help treat premenstrual syndrome, carpal tunnel syndrome, and hyperemesis gravidarum.
- Studies have shown that vitamin $B_6$ supplementation helps to improve cognitive function in the elderly.

## Benefits

- Vitamin $B_6$ can help improve mood disturbances in people with depression through two mechanisms: (1) promoting synthesis of serotonin, dopamine, and gamma-Aminobutyric acid (GABA) and (2) decreasing the levels of homocysteine, an amino acid linked to depression.
- Vitamin $B_6$ may help prevent and treat anemia.
- $B_6$ may also help prevent clogged arteries and thus reduce the risk of cardiovascular disease.

- Other studies have shown that this vitamin can reduce the risk of developing certain types of cancers, although the mechanisms involved are still not clear.

## Side Effects, Warnings, and Precautions

People who take high supplemental doses of vitamin $B_6$ (more than 2 grams per day) may experience some side effects such as numbness, tingling or burning in hands and feet, headache, and nausea. Taking high doses of vitamin $B_6$ for long periods can lead to significant nerve damage.

## Signs of Deficiency

Signs of vitamin $B_6$ deficiency include:

- Seizures
- Pruritic rash
- Confusion
- Depression
- Normocytic or microcytic anemia
- Cheilitis—inflammation of the lips
- Glossitis—inflammation of the tongue
- Immune response disturbances

Patients with mild deficiency may not develop symptoms and signs for many months or years. People treated with isoniazid (an anti-tuberculosis drug) should receive supplemental vitamin $B_6$ in order to prevent isoniazid-induced peripheral neuropathy. Individuals who consume plant-based diets, and patients who have autoimmune diseases, chronic renal failure,

and inflammatory bowel disease are also at risk of developing vitamin $B_6$ deficiency.

## How Much You Need

Vitamin $B_6$ cannot be stored in the body, and a daily supply is needed. The RDA is:

| AGE | MALE | FEMALE |
|---|---|---|
| 0–6 months | 0.1mg (AI not RDA)* | 0.1mg (AI not RDA)* |
| 7–12 months | 0.3mg (AI not RDA)* | 0.3mg (AI not RDA)* |
| 1–3 years | 0.5mg | 0.5mg |
| 4–8 years | 0.6mg | 0.6mg |
| 9–13 years | 1.0mg | 1.0mg |
| 14–18 years | 1.3mg | 1.2mg |
| 19–50 years | 1.3mg | 1.3mg |
| 51+ years | 1.7mg | 1.5mg |
| Pregnancy | – | 1.9mg |
| Lactation | – | 2.0mg |

* Adequate Intake amounts were developed for infants because there isn't sufficient evidence for a Recommended Daily Allowance (RDA).

## Tolerable Upper Intake Levels (Amount Per Day)

| AGE | MALE | FEMALE |
|---|---|---|
| 0–6 months | – | – |
| 7–12 months | – | – |
| 1–3 years | 30mg | 30mg |
| 4–8 years | 40mg | 40mg |
| 9–13 years | 60mg | 60mg |

| AGE | MALE | FEMALE |
|---|---|---|
| 14–18 years | 80mg | 80mg |
| 19+ years | 100mg | 100mg |
| Pregnancy | – | 100mg |
| Lactation | – | 100mg |

**Best Way to Consume**

The best dietary source of vitamin $B_6$ is animal foods. However, vitamin $B_6$ is sensitive to high temperatures and is partly destroyed during cooking. Milling and processing of whole-grain products removes a lot of this vitamin too.

## Natural Food Sources

| FOOD (SERVING SIZE) | VITAMIN $B_6$ (MG) |
|---|---|
| Chickpeas, canned, drained (1 cup) | 1.1 |
| Beef liver, pan fried (3 ounces) | 0.9 |
| Tuna, yellowfin, fresh, cooked (3 ounces) | 0.9 |
| Salmon, sockeye, cooked (3 ounces) | 0.6 |
| Potatoes, white, boiled, chopped (1 cup) | 0.4 |
| Banana, peeled (1 medium) | 0.4 |
| Turkey, meat only, roasted (3 ounces) | 0.4 |
| Ground beef, patty, 85% lean, broiled (3 ounces) | 0.3 |

## RECIPE

# Turkey Pita $B_6$ Boost  *Serves 1*

This mood-boosting recipe is packed with $B_6$ and will help you stay healthy and energized.

1 whole-grain pita pocket

1 leaf romaine lettuce

2 slices tomato

3 (1-ounce) slices natural, nitrate-free, low-sodium deli turkey

1 tablespoon Dijon mustard

3 sprigs fresh dill (or 2 teaspoons dried)

2 (1-ounce) slices provolone cheese

**PER SERVING**

*Calories: 500, Fat: 19g, Protein: 41g, Sodium: 1,705mg, Fiber: 6g, Carbohydrates: 40g, Sugar: 2g, $B_6$: 0.37mg*

Toast the pita and layer the rest of the ingredients in as you'd like. Enjoy!

# Vitamin B$_7$: Biotin

In 1942, biotin was discovered by Vincent du Vigneaud and his colleagues when they noticed that farm animals fed a certain diet developed biotin deficiency. Biotin is also called vitamin H because the *H* stands for *haar* and *haut*, which means "hair and skin" in German. Getting enough biotin, then, is important for healthy hair, skin, and many other functions. The good news is that since biotin is found in a wide range of foods, having a severe biotin deficiency is a rare occurrence. However, a mild biotin deficiency is actually quite common in pregnant women. Read on for tips on how to ensure you're meeting all of your biotin needs.

## Description

Similar to vitamin B$_5$, biotin is mainly involved with enabling enzymes (those little catalysts that help to foster a "chain reaction" of processes to occur in your body). The key point here is that a daily intake of vitamin B$_7$ is crucial for a wide range of processes to occur that impact cell development—and proper cell development is vital for your organ systems to function.

Biotin's main function is to enable the processes that are necessary for metabolizing fatty acids, glucose, and amino acids. If this all sounds very complicated, that's because these processes *are* very complex. Moreover, biotin acts as a cofactor for five enzymes with specific functions, termed carboxylases. In turn, each of these carboxylases exerts an influence on different biochemical actions in your body that affect your overall health.

Besides its foremost role in specific enzyme development, biotin also plays a key role in histone modifications, gene regulation, and cell signaling (instructing new cells in how to form).

Also, within the GI tract, other biochemicals produced by the body act on the consumed biotin, and it is then absorbed in the small intestine and stored in the liver.

## Role in the Body

- Biotin is required for the correct production of energy in your cells.
- It helps with the development of healthy, luminous hair and strong nails.

## Benefits

Besides its cellular energy–level benefit, biotin supplementation has been linked by a number of studies to healthier hair, nails, and skin. However, the scientific evidence remains inconclusive as to whether taking daily biotin supplements (without a diagnosed biotin deficiency) can actually improve hair, nails, and/or skin. Problematically, a recent research study concluded that the majority of biotin supplements marketed to consumers for the purpose of "better" hair, nails, or skin contain biotin amounts that *exceed* the Recommended Daily Allowance (RDA).

## Side Effects, Warnings, and Precautions

There are no particular warnings for a food intake of higher than the RDA of biotin. There are also no warnings for an intake of biotin supplements when ingested at no higher a dose than the RDA. However, pregnant women—who may require biotin supplements to treat a biotin deficiency—are advised not to take supplements at higher than the RDA.

Drug precautions exist regarding antibiotic medications (taken over a long period of time) and anti-seizure drugs, in that these have been linked to lower biotin levels in people who consume adequate biotin in their diets *and* in people who take biotin in supplements. Your biotin level may need to be monitored by a healthcare provider (e.g., physician or nurse practitioner) if you are taking high

doses of specific antibiotics or anti-seizure medications.

Also, several studies have concluded that diabetes interferes with biotin absorption.

## Signs of Deficiency

People suffering from severe malnutrition are most likely to experience a biotin deficiency. The most common symptoms of a biotin deficiency are:

- Fatigue
- Insomnia
- Dry or scaly skin
- Hair loss

People who have had bowel surgeries and those living with intestinal conditions like Crohn's disease may not be able to absorb enough biotin from foods. If you are in this group, taking a daily biotin supplement (as typically included in a B-complex vitamin pill) may be necessary.

People with chronic alcoholism are likely to experience a significant biotin (and other B vitamins) deficiency.

There is a rare inherited gene abnormality called Biotinidase (BTD) deficiency that disables biotin's capacity to be absorbed from food. In its mild form, this hereditary condition is associated with weak muscle tone, breathing problems, developmental delays, skin rashes, and/

or hair loss. According to the National Organization for Rare Disorders (NORD), children born with this disorder can be treated with biotin supplements.

## How Much You Need (RDA)

| AGE | MALE | FEMALE |
| --- | --- | --- |
| 0–12 months | 5–6mcg | 5–6mcg |
| 1–3 years | 8mcg | 8mcg |
| 4–8 years | 12mcg | 12mcg |
| 9–13 years | 20mcg | 20mcg |
| 14–18 years | 25mcg | 25mcg |
| 19+ years | 30mcg | 30mcg |
| Pregnancy | – | 30mcg |
| Lactation | – | 35mcg |

Taking biotin supplements at higher than the RDA is not recommended, as biotin in supplements has been found to interfere with lab-based results of blood tests. High doses of biotin supplements have been linked to false-positive test results for thyroid disorders.

## Best Way to Consume

For most people, the best way to consume biotin is in foods eaten as part of an overall healthy diet. Notably, biotin is absorbed at its optimal level when ingested with other B vitamins on a daily basis. Since it is excreted in urine, biotin needs to be ingested every day (along with the other B-complex vitamins). This vitamin is found in high amounts in organ meats, eggs, fish, and many vegetables (especially sweet potatoes). However, raw egg whites contain a protein that binds to biotin and interferes with your body's ability to absorb it.

## Natural Food Sources

| FOOD (SERVING SIZE) | BIOTIN (MCG) |
| --- | --- |
| Beef liver, cooked (3 ounces) | 30.8 |
| Egg, cooked (1 large) | 10 |
| Salmon, pink, canned in water, drained (3 ounces) | 5 |
| Tuna, canned in water, drained (3 ounces) | 0.6 |
| Spinach, boiled (½ cup) | 0.5 |
| Banana, peeled, sliced (½ cup) | 0.2 |

## Vegetable Omelet *Serves 1*

This is a simple yet nutrient-packed meal. This biotin-rich breakfast is guaranteed to make your day start off beautifully. Try it with some fresh herbs on top or switch up the veggies for variety.

| | | |
|---|---|---|
| 1 teaspoon extra-virgin olive oil | 1 tablespoon water | Pinch black pepper |
| ½ cup broccoli florets | ¼ teaspoon dried oregano | 1 ounce sun-dried tomatoes |
| ½ cup sliced mushrooms | Pinch cayenne pepper | |
| 2 large eggs, beaten | Pinch salt | |

**PER SERVING**

*Calories: 277, Fat: 14g, Protein: 19g, Sodium: 518mg, Fiber: 5g, Carbohydrates: 21g, Sugar: 13g*

1 Heat oil in a medium skillet over medium heat. Add broccoli and mushrooms and cook until veggies are tender, about 3–5 minutes.

2 In a small bowl, combine eggs with water, oregano, cayenne, salt, and black pepper.

3 Pour egg mixture over the vegetables in the pan, add sun-dried tomatoes, and cook until the bottom is solid.

4 Flip over and cook 5 more minutes or until eggs are solid. Serve.

# Vitamin B₉: Folate

Vitamin B$_9$, or folate—also called folic acid—is probably best known for its role in helping ensure proper formation of the spine in babies during early pregnancy. The extraordinary discovery of this vitamin was due to the pioneering research of a brilliant female scientist in the 1920s named Lucy Wills. Dr. Wills attended the first medical school in England to allow women to enter. After completing medical school, she lived and traveled the world, making her breakthrough discovery that led to what is now known as folate while she was living and working in Bombay, India. This landmark discovery has helped ensure the delivery of countless healthy babies and the prevention of serious birth defects, another tremendous public health success.

## Description

Folate has numerous key functions. It is essential for normal cell growth and division in the human body and particularly for proper spine and brain development in babies. The name "folate" comes from the Latin word for "leaf," *folium*, because it is naturally present in vegetables (especially green, leafy vegetables). Folate is the name for the vitamin that occurs naturally in foods, while folic acid is the synthetic version that is in supplements and fortified foods.

Proper absorption of vitamin B$_{12}$ is dependent upon an adequate intake of folate. All B-complex vitamins need to be ingested in acceptable amounts in the daily diet for each to function properly, but this is especially true in the case of vitamin B$_{12}$ and folate, since these function together in the enzymatic methylation process. Folate is essential for red blood cell (RBC) formation and human cell growth. Folate works with B$_{12}$ to create RBCs and prevent anemia. Like any true partnership, these two vitamins must be in balance for the proper formation of blood cells plus a few other important functions.

## Role in the Body

- Folate plays a critical role in the body's biochemical process of methylation, which is necessary for DNA synthesis; detoxification; and energy production.
- It plays a key role in the metabolism of nucleic acid precursors (affecting DNA integrity) and the metabolism of amino acids (such as homocysteine).
- A folate deficiency can result in megaloblastic anemia. This type of anemia

is the consequence of immature RBC formation. Brain damage can result if this is left untreated and becomes severe.

- In combination with vitamins $B_{12}$ and $B_6$, folate curbs abnormally high levels of blood homocysteine, which are linked to heart disease.

## Benefits

- **Improves brain health:** Consumption of a folate-rich diet is essential to preventing neurological and brain-related disorders. As stated in *Psychology Today* in 2016, folate is necessary for creation of the brain's neurotransmitters and for cellular detoxification, as well as for DNA formation and the proper development of the nervous system.
- **Improves mood:** Low levels of folate can negatively affect serotonin synthesis, which plays a role in depression and mood regulation. Having adequate folate levels seems to improve and prevent mood disorders like depression. In fact, many researchers have suggested that supplemental folate be considered as a treatment for depression, though more studies are needed in this area.
- **Reduces cancer risk:** A study published in the *American Journal of Epidemiology* in 2011 showed that adequate folate intake from food sources may reduce breast cancer risk in premenopausal women, and that women with low intake had higher rates of breast cancer.
- **Promotes heart health:** Research indicates that folate is likely heart protective and can help to reduce risk of heart disease.
- **Contributes to having a healthy baby:** Folic acid helps ensure delivery of a healthy baby and lowers the risk of brain and spine defects.

## Side Effects, Warnings, and Precautions

Taking high doses of folic acid supplements or eating too many fortified foods can cause excitability, sleep disorders, and seizures. There's emerging concern among researchers that getting too much synthetic folic acid (not folate) can also potentially increase risk of cancer. It is recommended that if you are not of childbearing age you should get folate from food sources exclusively.

Some medications negatively interact with folic acid. These include methotrexate (used to treat cancer and autoimmune disorders), anti-epileptic medications (e.g., phenytoin), and sulfasalazine (used in the treatment of ulcerative colitis).

Lab test results show that pernicious anemia (a vitamin $B_{12}$ deficiency) can be masked by a high daily intake of folic acid, so it is generally recommended that people who may have pernicious anemia not take folic acid supplements, so that a conclusive diagnosis can be achieved.

One consequence of an inability to absorb folate (resulting in a folate deficiency) is a higher risk for cognitive impairment in aging. In a 2005 study published in *The American Journal of Clinical Nutrition*, folate deficiency was found to be linked to dementia.

## Signs of Deficiency

Symptoms of folate deficiency can be subtle (e.g., fatigue and dizziness) and can mimic other health disorders. However, a more severe deficiency in daily folate intake can lead to folate-deficiency anemia. Signs of more severe folate deficiency include:

- Fatigue
- Irritability
- Cognitive impairments
- Shortness of breath

People with poor folate absorption typically experience a high degree of fatigue and malaise, as well as RBC-related anemia.

Excessive alcohol use (i.e., alcoholism) and chronic smoking have been linked to decreased absorption of folate, as have inflammatory bowel diseases (e.g.,

Crohn's disease) and colon resection surgeries.

People who have intestinal disorders that interfere with nutrient absorption can develop a folate deficiency, despite an adequate daily intake of folate-containing foods. And some people are genetically predisposed to an inability to absorb folic acid.

## How Much You Need (RDA)

| AGE | MALE | FEMALE |
| --- | --- | --- |
| 0–6 months | 65mcg (AI not RDA)* | 65mcg (AI not RDA)* |
| 7–12 months | 80mcg (AI not RDA)* | 80mcg (AI not RDA)* |
| 1–3 years | 150mcg | 150mcg |
| 4–8 years | 200mcg | 200mcg |
| 9–13 years | 300mcg | 300mcg |
| 14–18 years | 400mcg | 400mcg |
| 19+ years | 400mcg | 400mcg |
| Pregnancy | – | 600mcg |
| Lactation | – | 500mcg |

* Adequate Intake amounts were developed for infants because there isn't sufficient evidence for a Recommended Daily Allowance (RDA).

Since so many people do not get the optimal amount of folate through their diet, the Centers for Disease Control and Prevention (CDC) recommends that women of reproductive age take 400mcg of folic acid in a supplement each day. This is because around half of pregnancies in the US are not planned and the major birth defects that folate can help to prevent occur before most women even know they are pregnant—at around three to four weeks after conception. Ensuring there's optimal folate can help ensure a healthy baby.

**Best Way to Consume**

Eating a balanced diet is the best way to consume vitamin $B_9$. The best way to ensure consumption of this vitamin is to include green vegetables and fruit daily. Many other foods are fortified, such as folic acid–fortified cereal and grain products. Meanwhile, for people with intestinal disorders that negatively affect nutrient absorption from food, or for people who need a higher amount, like women of childbearing age, a high-quality supplement will likely be needed.

## Natural Food Sources

| FOOD (SERVING SIZE) | FOLATE (MCG) |
| --- | --- |
| Beef liver, braised (3 ounces) | 215 |
| Spinach, boiled (½ cup) | 131 |
| Avocado, peeled, pitted, cubed (½ cup) | 59 |
| Green peas, frozen, boiled (½ cup) | 47 |
| Wheatgerm (2 tablespoons) | 40 |
| Peanuts, dry roasted (1 ounce) | 27 |
| Banana, peeled (1 medium) | 24 |

# Wild Rice Detox Bowl *Serves 1*

Wild rice is packed with nutrients and tastes very unique. Combined with vegetables and lentils, it makes a perfectly balanced meal that will boost your folate stores.

½ tablespoon extra-virgin olive oil

1 clove garlic, minced

¼ cup chopped green onion

½ teaspoon turmeric

1 small carrot, shredded

1 cup chopped spinach

½ cup precooked or canned lentils, rinsed

Pinch salt

½ cup cooked wild rice

¼ medium avocado, peeled, pitted, and sliced

**PER SERVING**
*Calories: 353, Fat: 12g, Protein: 15g, Sodium: 356mg, Fiber: 15g, Carbohydrates: 50g, Sugar: 6g, Folate: 313mcg*

1  Heat oil in a medium skillet over medium heat. Add garlic, onion, turmeric, and carrot. Cook 3 minutes.
2  Add spinach and lentils and cook another 2–3 minutes. Add salt as needed.
3  Serve lentil mixture over the wild rice and top with avocado. Enjoy!

# Vitamin B$_{12}$

Vitamin B$_{12}$ is known as the energy vitamin. It is a powerhouse that helps the body to make DNA and red blood cells. Vitamin B$_{12}$ is the largest of the B-complex vitamins, and it helps your nerves to fire quickly and your red blood cells to fill up with life-giving oxygen. Vitamin B$_{12}$ also aids in DNA formation (that encodes genes). Like other B-complex vitamins (as well as vitamin C), it is a water-soluble vitamin, so not much B$_{12}$ is stored in the body, and you have to ingest it daily to ensure optimal levels. According to a 2017 article in *American Family Physician*, vitamin B$_{12}$ deficiency in the US and UK is around 6 percent in people under sixty years of age and almost 20 percent among those older than sixty. In some countries in Latin America, Asia, and Africa deficiency can be as high as 70 percent. Fortunately, there are plenty of nourishing foods you can start including in your diet right away to boost your levels.

## Description

Did you know that B$_{12}$ is made by bacteria both in your gut and also in the digestive tracts of many animals? This is why animal sources are the highest in B$_{12}$, with only seaweed as a potential non-animal source. The symptoms of low B$_{12}$ are quite nonspecific and generalized, such as fatigue, weakness, and depression—and it's not something that's routinely tested for at most doctor's visits, even though B$_{12}$ can be evaluated via an easy blood test. Many experts recommend that individuals get their B$_{12}$ levels checked at least once, as numerous different factors can cause deficiency, even in those who eat plenty of animal products. Various medical conditions as well as parasites, gut disorders, strict vegan diets, certain medicines, and alcohol can all decrease B$_{12}$ levels significantly.

## Role in the Body

Vitamin B$_{12}$ is normally involved in:

- Fatty acid synthesis
- Energy production
- DNA synthesis

People who are unable to properly absorb vitamin B$_{12}$ may feel fatigued and may experience cognitive deficits (such as memory problems) or neurological symptoms (such as a tingling and/or numbness in hands and feet).

## Benefits

The most important benefit of adequate vitamin B$_{12}$ intake is that it prevents pernicious anemia symptoms (also termed megaloblastic anemia). People who have had a portion of their stomach or intestines removed, have a thyroid disorder, or have an autoimmune disorder (such as type 1 diabetes) are at higher risk of pernicious anemia, so ensuring an adequate intake of vitamin $B_{12}$ in their daily diet may be beneficial to avoid a deficiency and its symptoms.

Study findings published in *The New England Journal of Medicine* in 2014 showed that people taking antidepressants who experienced a return of depressive symptoms reported a lessening of their depression following $B_{12}$ supplementation. Findings published in other medical journals have also suggested that $B_{12}$ supplementation may lessen depression and anxiety symptoms in patients who have been diagnosed with a $B_{12}$ deficiency.

## Side Effects, Warnings, and Precautions

Folate (folic acid in supplements) is often prescribed along with vitamin $B_{12}$ to treat pernicious anemia, but—as previously mentioned—too much folate can promote $B_{12}$ deficiency. Vitamin $B_{12}$ supplements should not be taken by people who are allergic to them, have a genetic condition called optic atrophy, or have been diagnosed with polycythemia (a blood cancer).

Since vitamin $B_{12}$ crosses the placenta in pregnancy (and also enters breast milk), pregnant and lactating women should only take vitamin $B_{12}$ supplements under their doctor's supervision.

## Signs of Deficiency

Signs of deficiency can include:

- Weakness
- Fatigue
- Confusion
- Constipation
- Loss of appetite

Deficiency is also associated with memory loss, depression, and tongue soreness. In severe cases, it can cause nerve damage and must be treated immediately.

A vitamin $B_{12}$ deficiency can result from not ingesting enough $B_{12}$, a health disorder causing insufficient absorption, or taking certain drugs that interfere with vitamin $B_{12}$ absorption. In general, people sixty and older have a higher risk of developing a $B_{12}$ deficiency than younger people. One reason is that secretion of hydrochloric acid (HCl) in the stomach decreases in aging—and this is necessary for proper digestion of nutrients.

People who have experienced the following are also more likely to develop a vitamin $B_{12}$ deficiency:

- Autoimmune disorders affecting the gut (such as celiac disease or Crohn's disease)
- Gastric bypass or other gastrointestinal surgery
- Pernicious anemia
- Parasite or worm infections
- Regularly consuming certain medications, such as those used to treat acid reflux or heartburn, metformin (a diabetes medication), or hormone replacement therapy (HRT)

Since vegetarians and vegans consume few to no animal products they are also at higher risk of vitamin $B_{12}$ deficiency.

## How Much You Need

| AGE | MALE | FEMALE |
| --- | --- | --- |
| 0–6 months | 0.4mcg (AI not RDA)* | 0.4mcg (AI not RDA)* |
| 7–12 months | 0.5mcg (AI not RDA)* | 0.5mcg (AI not RDA)* |
| 1–3 years | 0.9mcg | 0.9mcg |
| 4–8 years | 1.2mcg | 1.2mcg |
| 9–13 years | 1.8mcg | 1.8mcg |
| 14+ years | 2.4mcg | 2.4mcg |
| Pregnancy | – | 2.6mcg |
| Lactation | – | 2.8mcg |

* Adequate Intake amounts were developed for infants because there isn't sufficient evidence for a Recommended Daily Allowance (RDA).

## Best Way to Consume

Animal products such as eggs, dairy, meat, fish, and poultry are the best sources of vitamin $B_{12}$. According to the Mayo Clinic, if you follow a vegan diet, you may be especially susceptible to a vitamin $B_{12}$ deficiency, as plant foods do not contain vitamin $B_{12}$. The ideal way to consume vitamin $B_{12}$ is in foods, but this may not be possible if you are unable to absorb $B_{12}$ for any reason.

Many fortified breakfast cereals in the US, Canada, and Europe contain vitamin $B_{12}$, and for those who don't eat animal products, vitamin supplements are another way to ensure an adequate intake. For people who cannot absorb enough vitamin $B_{12}$ orally, intramuscular injections of $B_{12}$ can be administered by a physician.

## Natural Food Sources

| FOOD (SERVING SIZE) | $B_{12}$ (MCG) |
| --- | --- |
| Clams, cooked (3 ounces) | 84.1 |
| Beef liver, cooked (3½ ounces) | 70.7 |
| Trout, rainbow, wild, cooked (3 ounces) | 5.4 |
| Salmon, sockeye, cooked (3 ounces) | 4.8 |
| Tuna, light, canned in water, drained (3 ounces) | 2.5 |
| Milk, low-fat (1 cup) | 1.2 |

## RECIPE

# Protein Scramble with Super Greens  *Serves 1*

This protein scramble is easy to make and will fuel your morning with $B_{12}$, healthy protein, heart-healthy fats, detoxing fiber, and tons of phytonutrients and antioxidants from the super greens and anti-inflammatory spices. It's perfect for mornings when you have to be on top of your game or just want to feel fueled.

2 teaspoons extra-virgin olive oil

½ cup shredded kale

½ cup spinach

¼ cup chopped onion

2 large eggs

2 tablespoons low-fat milk (or plant-based milk)

⅛ teaspoon paprika powder

⅛ cup shredded mozzarella cheese

Pinch salt

Pinch black pepper

**PER SERVING**
*Calories: 301, Fat: 21g, Protein: 18g, Sodium: 558mg, Fiber: 1g, Carbohydrates: 8g, Sugar: 3g, $B_{12}$: 1.3mcg*

1 In a medium cast-iron or nonstick skillet over medium heat, warm oil. Add kale, spinach, and onion and sauté 4–5 minutes or until onion becomes translucent and greens wilt.

2 While veggies are cooking, beat eggs in a small bowl with milk and paprika.

3 Add egg mixture to skillet and gently mix with vegetables. Cook until egg mixture cooks all the way through, about 3–4 minutes.

4 Top with cheese, salt, and pepper and enjoy!

# Vitamin C

Remarkably, vitamin C, also known as ascorbic acid, can be synthesized in almost all mammals except humans. We don't have the enzyme required to make it. In 1927, vitamin C was discovered by Hungarian biochemist and humanitarian Albert Szent-Györgyi when he realized that the body needs ascorbic acid to use macronutrients (carbohydrates, fats, and proteins) more efficiently. Dr. Szent-Györgyi went on to receive the Nobel prize for his scientific work and discovery of vitamin C.

## Description

Arguably one of the most well-known and popular vitamins, vitamin C is ubiquitous, as are misconceptions about it. Did you know that taking vitamin C as a supplement may cause it to be absorbed and used less efficiently in your body than if you get it from whole foods? This is likely due to the fact that the best natural sources of vitamin C, fruits and vegetables, are also high in many other beneficial compounds and nutrients, such as numerous phytochemicals, which work to boost its action. Some of these compounds haven't even been identified yet, but as more research is done, it's become more and more clear that they play a synergistic role in how vitamins are absorbed and used in the body. Nature is remarkable, and simply isolating one compound, like vitamin C, usually doesn't work as well as having the whole package of nutrients working together. Think of it like a symphony: While a single instrument sounds lovely on its own, the combination of all the instruments playing together is truly magnificent.

## Role in the Body

Vitamin C helps to build and repair all tissues in your body, making it a critically important nutrient. For example, it helps:

- Cuts and wounds heal faster
- Bones and cartilage stay strong
- Your immune system fight off disease and infections more efficiently

Vitamin C is also essential in the formation of collagen, which is the main protein in the body, helping to make up all of your tissues, skin, and muscle. Collagen production in the body starts to decrease around age twenty-five, which can cause skin and tissue aging. In order to boost collagen and keep levels as high as possible, vitamin C is important.

## Benefits

Some of vitamin C's many benefits include:

- It is essential for overall body repair and growth.
- It helps delay or prevent heart diseases, cancer, and the common cold.
- It contributes to eye health.
- Consumption of vitamin C with iron enhances the absorption of iron in the small intestine.
- As an antioxidant, vitamin C works as a reducing agent and neutralizes free radicals in the body, which means that it slows down and prevents cellular damage from free radicals.
- Vitamin C helps increase production of white blood cells, which are the protectors of our body, slaying harmful foreign invaders like cold and flu viruses and bad bacteria.
- It can help reduce risk of chronic diseases.
- Vitamin C helps prevent iron deficiency by converting plant-based iron into a form that's more easily taken up by the body, which is important for everyone, but especially for vegans and vegetarians, who typically consume less iron, as they do not eat meat.

## Side Effects, Warnings, and Precautions

Vitamin C absorption decreases with increased intake, meaning if your vitamin C intake is more than 1 gram, your absorption is less than 50 percent. Another precaution about vitamin C is that it is sensitive to heat, light, oxidation, and alkaline solutions. It is more stable in acidic solutions.

Taking high doses of vitamin C can cause gastrointestinal problems like abdominal pain and diarrhea due to bacterial metabolism of unabsorbed vitamin C in the colon. If you have a history of renal problems, high dosage of vitamin C might increase the risk of kidney stones.

## Signs of Deficiency

Scurvy, the disease associated with vitamin C deficiency, was first seen among British sailors due to lack of fresh vegetables and fruits. After the discovery, sailors started taking limes with them when they went out to sea, garnering them the nickname "limey."

In developed countries, vitamin C deficiency is rare, but it can still occur in people with limited food variety, smokers, and "passive" smokers.

Symptoms of scurvy appear when the total pool of vitamin C in the body drops below 300 milligrams. Scurvy is rare though still present in developed countries. It can occur among smokers and the elderly with poor diet coupled with alcoholism or drug abuse.

## How Much You Need

| AGE | MALE | FEMALE |
| --- | --- | --- |
| 0–6 months | 40mg (AI not RDA)* | 40mg (AI not RDA)* |
| 7–12 months | 50mg (AI not RDA)* | 50mg (AI not RDA)* |
| 1–3 years | 15mg | 15mg |
| 4–8 years | 25mg | 25mg |
| 9–13 years | 45mg | 45mg |
| 14–18 years | 75mg | 65mg |
| 19+ years | 90mg | 75mg |
| Pregnancy | – | 85mg |
| Lactation | – | 120mg |

* Adequate Intake amounts were developed for infants because there isn't sufficient evidence for a Recommended Daily Allowance (RDA).

In addition, smokers need 35 milligrams per day more vitamin C than nonsmokers.

## Best Way to Consume

Vitamin C is absorbed throughout the small intestine. Research indicates that bioavailability of vitamin C is improved when it's eaten in the form of fruits and vegetables. Since the body tightly controls the blood levels of this vitamin, taking high doses (anything over 1 gram) will just put extra stress on the kidneys as they excrete the extra amounts—and absorption will be greatly decreased. If you want to boost your vitamin C, instead of a supplement, choose brightly colored fruits and vegetables and try to eat at least two fruits and four to six vegetables each day.

## Natural Food Sources

| FOOD (SERVING SIZE) | VITAMIN C (MG) |
| --- | --- |
| Guava (1 medium) | 126 |
| Bell pepper, red, chopped (½ cup) | 95 |
| Papaya (1 small) | 95 |
| Kiwifruit (1 large) | 85 |
| Orange (1 medium) | 70 |
| Bell pepper, green, chopped (½ cup) | 60 |
| Strawberries, sliced (½ cup) | 49 |

| FOOD (SERVING SIZE) | VITAMIN C (MG) |
| --- | --- |
| Broccoli, chopped, boiled, drained (½ cup) | 39 |
| Tomato juice, canned (6 ounces) | 33 |
| Cauliflower, raw or cooked (½ cup) | 26 |

## RECIPE

# Almond and Goji Berry Morning Smoothie *Serves 1*

Filled with vitamin C, antioxidants, and some plant-based protein, this fruity smoothie will give you a scrumptious boost after your morning workout!

1½ tablespoons dried goji berries

¾ cup soy milk

¼ cup frozen mango chunks

½ medium frozen banana, peeled

½ medium orange, peeled and seeds removed

1 cup spinach

Ice cubes, as needed

**PER SERVING**
*Calories: 202, Fat: 4g, Protein: 8g, Sodium: 115mg, Fiber: 6g, Carbohydrates: 37g, Sugar: 24g, Vitamin C: 64mg*

Add all ingredients to a blender and blend until smooth. Add more ice if needed to achieve desired consistency. Serve immediately.

# Calcium

Calcium is the most abundant mineral in the human body and it's what helps you to have strong bones and teeth. Calcium is found everywhere in nature. It's the fifth-most abundant element in the earth's crust and is commonly found in many rocks like limestone or gypsum. It's most known for its role in our bone structure, but it has a plethora of other functions inside your body. Despite how important it is, some estimates show that only 10–15 percent of teenage girls and women over fifty are meeting their needs! The numbers are slightly better for teen boys and men over fifty— around 20 percent meet their needs through diet, but that's still way too low. Read on for easy ways to get more calcium from your diet.

## Description

Getting calcium while you are young is critical. Our bones continue building and getting stronger until we are around twenty to twenty-five years old, so you need to eat a calcium-rich diet to ensure your bones and teeth are able to become as dense as possible. After age twenty-five, bone density, or the strength of the bones, starts to decline. If you don't get enough calcium in these early years, it can put you at risk for osteoporosis (accelerated bone loss and weakening) as you get older. But getting enough calcium after the age of twenty-five is important too. Calcium plays a role in all kinds of signaling and communication pathways in the body, so it's critical to survival. If there isn't enough calcium in the blood, your body will pull it from the bones to maintain homeostasis, or balance, in your system. It's a complex and remarkable mechanism that makes sure calcium levels stay constant at all times, even at the cost of your bone health.

Since there are many foods that are rich in calcium, getting enough of it through foods shouldn't be too much of a challenge, if you are eating a healthy, balanced diet. If you eat some animal products, like dairy and fish, you're probably getting enough. Vegans need to plan their meals more carefully, but there are some plant sources too.

## Role in the Body

Calcium plays several roles in the body, including:

- **Bone and tooth formation and structure:** Bones and teeth contain 99 percent of the calcium in the body. Bones are breaking down and remodeling all the time, and calcium is the main mineral required for this process to function properly.

- **Nerve signaling:** With all the signals firing in the brain, calcium plays an important role in balancing brain activities.
- **Blood clot formation:** The 1 percent of calcium that is not in bone is found in the blood and works with vitamin K to form blood clots.
- **Muscle function:** Inside your muscles, calcium binds to the fibers actin and myosin and helps facilitate the interaction between them to change position and allow the muscles to contract.

## Benefits
Benefits of calcium include:

- **Strong bones and full height potential:** Calcium increases the quality and density of bones and is needed during childhood to ensure that you reach your full growth in height.
- **Possible protection against diabetes:** Studies have demonstrated that appropriate calcium and vitamin D intake can help you maintain a healthy body weight and BMI, and decrease the risk of type 2 diabetes.
- **Maintenance of normal blood pressure:** Several clinical trials have shown that increased calcium consumption is inversely associated with risk of hypertension and high blood pressure.
- **Possible protection against cancer:** It's been shown that consuming the recommended amount of calcium may lower the chances of colorectal and breast cancers.

## Side Effects, Warnings, and Precautions
Getting too much calcium (unlikely if you're just getting it from foods) can carry risks. Consuming over 2,500 milligrams daily from supplements can increase the chances of kidney stones and kidney damage, and it may reduce the body's ability to absorb other minerals like magnesium, zinc, and iron.

## Signs of Deficiency
Signs of deficiency can include:

- **Weak bones leading to osteoporosis:** If you do not get enough calcium, your bones will not grow properly and can become weak and brittle and more likely to fracture.
- **Tooth erosion:** Healthy teeth require enough calcium to heal and stay healthy and erosion-free.
- **Muscle cramps:** Low calcium levels in the blood might result in muscle cramps, a condition also known as tetany.

## How Much You Need (RDA)

| AGE | MALE | FEMALE |
| --- | --- | --- |
| 0–12 months | 200–260mg (AI not RDA)* | 200–260mg (AI not RDA)* |
| 1–3 years | 700mg | 700mg |
| 4–8 years | 1,000mg | 1,000mg |
| 9–18 years | 1,300mg | 1,300mg |
| 19–50 years | 1,300mg | 1,300mg |
| 51–70 years | 1,000mg | 1,000mg |
| 71+ years | 1,200mg | 1,200mg |
| Pregnancy | – | 1,000mg |
| Lactation | – | 1,000mg |

* Adequate Intake amounts were developed for infants because there isn't sufficient evidence for a Recommended Daily Allowance (RDA).

## Tolerable Upper Intake Levels (Amount Per Day)

| AGE | MALE | FEMALE |
| --- | --- | --- |
| 0–6 months | 1,000mg | 1,000mg |
| 7–12 months | 1,500mg | 1,500mg |
| 1–8 years | 2,500mg | 2,500mg |
| 9–18 years | 3,000mg | 3,000mg |
| 19–50 years | 2,500mg | 2,500mg |
| 51+ years | 2,000mg | 2,000mg |
| Pregnancy | – | 2,500mg |
| Lactation | – | 2,500mg |

## Best Way to Consume

Calcium requires the help of vitamin D to be absorbed. Combining foods rich in calcium and vitamin D can help ensure you're optimizing your levels of both.

One of the best sources for calcium and vitamin D is canned fish, like sardines, herring, and mackerel. The soft bones are edible and contain a ton of calcium. The small fish are best because they contain less mercury and environmental contaminants and more calcium than bigger fish, like tuna. Always make sure to check sources like Seafood Watch for the most up-to-date information on which fish are the most environmentally sustainable. You can also look for certifications like the MSC (Marine Stewardship Council) seal for wild fish and the BAP (Best Aquaculture Practices) seal for farmed fish on labels to be certain that environmental, social, and economic factors of fish sourcing are considered.

If you're a vegan or vegetarian, there are plenty of sources of calcium, like most dark leafy greens. Keep in mind that you'll need to consume a bit more of them to meet your needs than people who consume them in addition to animal products.

## Natural Food Sources

| FOOD (SERVING SIZE) | CALCIUM (MG) |
| --- | --- |
| Plain yogurt, low-fat (8 ounces) | 415 |
| Mozzarella, part-skim (1½ ounces) | 333 |
| Sardines, canned in oil, with bones, drained (3 ounces) | 325 |
| Milk, nonfat (8 ounces) | 299 |
| Soy milk, calcium-fortified (8 ounces) | 299 |
| Salmon, pink, canned in oil, with bones, drained (3 ounces) | 261 |
| Chia seeds (1 ounce) | 179 |
| Tofu, soft, made with calcium sulfate, cubed (½ cup) | 138 |
| Turnip, green, fresh, boiled (½ cup) | 99 |
| Kale, fresh, cooked (1 cup) | 94 |
| Collard greens, raw (1 cup) | 84 |
| Okra, cooked (1 cup) | 82 |
| Chinese cabbage, bok choy, raw (1 cup) | 74 |
| Spinach, raw (½ cup) | 29 |
| Broccoli, raw, chopped (½ cup) | 21 |

# Turnip, Mackerel, and Greens Casserole  *Serves 2*

This recipe is packed with dietary sources of calcium. Mackerel, greens, and dairy are some of the best ways to consume calcium. This is another good recipe to make a big batch of and have on hand during the week.

½ cup almond milk

2 large eggs

2 teaspoons dried sage

2 teaspoons dried thyme

Pinch salt

Pinch black pepper

2 teaspoons extra-virgin olive oil

2 large turnips, sliced into thin rounds

1 (15-ounce) can wild mackerel, drained

½ cup chopped kale

¼ cup grated Parmesan cheese

**PER SERVING**
*Calories: 522, Fat: 23g, Protein: 54g, Sodium: 1,287mg, Fiber: 4g, Carbohydrates: 19g, Sugar: 11g, Calcium: 757mg*

1  Preheat oven to 360°F.

2  In a medium bowl, whisk together almond milk, eggs, sage, thyme, salt, and pepper.

3  Oil a medium baking dish and add half of the turnips, then add a layer of mackerel, then kale, followed by another layer of remaining turnips.

4  Pour milk and egg mixture over vegetables and mackerel, top with cheese, and bake about 25 minutes or until solid and golden brown on top.

# Chloride

Chloride is not a nutrient that you hear about very often, but it's actually one of the major minerals that is also an electrolyte (along with sodium and potassium). Electrolytes help to transmit nerve and electrical signals inside the body. They also have the very important role of regulating fluid balance inside and outside of your cells. Chlorine and chloride are closely related but are not the same. Chlorine, in its pure (elemental) form, is a greenish-colored gas that bonds with other minerals, such as sodium. So, regular table salt is sodium chloride, which is made up of about 60 percent chloride and 40 percent sodium, by weight.

## Description

Chloride is essential for survival. Deficiency is almost nonexistent in developed countries because of the wide availability of salt (which is almost half sodium and half chloride). Chloride is toxic when it's in the gaseous chlorine form, but when it's combined with another mineral like sodium, it's used by the body for numerous key metabolic functions.

You can think of chloride as sodium's better half; they are usually found together, but chloride tends to cause much less harm than its partner in crime.

Chloride also joins with other minerals to make compounds that can treat various conditions. There's magnesium chloride and potassium chloride, which are used to boost magnesium and potassium if they are low in the blood.

## Role in the Body

- **Fluid balance in the body:** As one of the three key electrolyte minerals, chloride helps maintain fluid balance inside and outside the cells.
- **Formation of stomach acid:** HCl, KCl, and NaCl are all components of stomach acid. Do you see the Cl there? That's chloride. Stomach acid is a potent digestive aid and helps break down food in the stomach.
- **Assists the nervous system with electrical impulse transmission:** Along with other electrolyte molecules, chloride helps create electrical signals so our muscles can contract and relax.

## Benefits

- Digestion and breakdown of food
- Hydration and fluid balance
- Nerve signal functioning

## Side Effects, Warnings, and Precautions

Our bodies eliminate excess chloride primarily through the kidneys, while creating urine. A very small amount is also eliminated in the stool and by sweating. High levels of chloride are rare but can occur when your body loses a lot of water and your blood becomes very concentrated with chloride, or if you take in too much salt. Many studies suggest that very high levels of chloride in the blood, called hyperchloremia, can even cause kidney injury. Also, high levels of chloride can throw off the acid-base balance in your body, causing a lower pH. This can affect a lot of different processes, like how your neurotransmitters function, how your blood vessels contract, and even how your blood clots.

## Signs of Deficiency

Chloride deficiency is quite rare, and like other electrolyte deficiencies, it can be caused by large losses of fluids, like those due to significant vomiting, diarrhea, and so on. In severe cases it can lead to a life-threatening state called alkalosis, a condition in which the blood pH level is higher than normal. Additionally, some drugs, like diuretics, are another factor that might cause low blood chloride levels.

Signs of deficiency can include:

- Weakness
- Nausea and vomiting
- Convulsions
- Coma

## How Much You Need

There is no RDA for chloride, but there is an Adequate Intake (AI). When there is not enough scientific evidence to establish RDA intake for a nutrient, AI provides a value based on experiments and observations to ensure nutritional adequacy.

| AGE | MALE | FEMALE |
| --- | --- | --- |
| 0–6 months | 0.18g | 0.18g |
| 7–12 months | 0.57g | 0.57g |
| 1–3 years | 1.5g | 1.5g |
| 4–8 years | 1.9g | 2.9g |
| 9–13 years | 2.3g | 2.3g |
| 14–18 years | 2.3g | 2.3g |
| 19–50 years | 2.3g | 2.3g |
| 51+ years | 1.8–2.0g | 1.8–2.0g |
| Pregnancy | – | 2.3g |
| Lactation | – | 2.3g |

## Upper Limit (Amount Per Day)

| AGE | MALE | FEMALE |
| --- | --- | --- |
| 0–12 months | Not established | Not established |
| 1–3 years | 2.3g | 2.3g |
| 4–8 years | 2.9g | 2.9g |
| 9–13 years | 3.4g | 3.4g |
| 14–18 years | 3. 6g | 3. 6g |
| 19–50 years | 3.6g | 3.6g |
| 51+ years | 3.6g | 3.6g |
| Pregnancy | – | 3.6g |
| Lactation | – | 3.6g |

## Best Way to Consume

The most common way to get chloride is by eating salt. Chloride is naturally present in ocean water, so plants like seaweed will also have chloride. Most people overconsume salt, so it's easy to get plenty of chloride without even trying! Some foods that naturally contain it are listed in the next section.

## Natural Food Sources

Chloride is not a nutrient commonly measured in food sources. The following foods are known to naturally have some chloride, but the amount is not typically measured.

- Salt
- Seaweed
- Oysters
- Celery
- Tomatoes
- Boiled eggs
- Olives in brine

# Sushi Bowl with Wild Rice *Serves 1*

Seaweed is an excellent source of chloride. This delicious bowl is the perfect way to optimize your stores.

½ cup cooked wild rice

2 ounces sushi-grade tuna

1 small head bok choy, chopped

1 small carrot, shredded

¼ medium avocado, peeled, pitted, and sliced

1 sheet nori, shredded

1 tablespoon pickled ginger

1 tablespoon low-sodium soy sauce

1 teaspoon sesame seeds

1 teaspoon wasabi paste

**PER SERVING**
*Calories: 408, Fat: 12g,
Protein: 34g, Sodium:
1,337mg, Fiber: 15g,
Carbohydrates: 50g,
Sugar: 13g*

1  Assemble rice, tuna, bok choy, carrot, avocado, nori, ginger, and soy sauce in a medium bowl.
2  Top with sesame seeds and wasabi as desired. Enjoy!

# Choline

Choline is the new kid on the block when it comes to essential nutrients. Even though it was discovered in 1862, the Institute of Medicine only started calling choline an essential nutrient in 1998. Deficiency in choline, like deficiency in any other essential vitamin or nutrient, will lead to disease and, if not treated, ultimately death. Choline is totally unique. It's neither a vitamin nor a mineral but rather is a compound similar in structure to some of the B vitamins. We are still learning about its role in the body and how much we need, but we do know it has a few fascinating functions, as you'll see in this entry.

## Description

Although it's easy to find choline-rich foods, most people aren't eating a proper amount of this essential nutrient. Low levels of choline can raise the risk of pregnancy complications, liver damage, and weakness in muscles. Your liver makes a small amount of choline, but that is not enough to meet your daily needs. People with liver problems or damage often make even less choline than the average person. Interestingly, choline production is linked to another vitamin, folate. When you have enough folate (a good source is leafy greens), your body can make more choline.

## Role in the Body

- **Brain development:** Especially important during pregnancy, choline helps with the fetus's brain and nervous system formation.
- **Liver function:** As more research emerges, we're learning that choline is needed for a healthy liver and prevention of fatty liver disease.
- **Metabolism:** It's essential for fat transport and metabolism. Insufficient amounts of choline can interfere with weight loss and lead to a buildup of unhealthy fats.
- **Cell structure and communication:** Cells send messages to each other via little "messenger" molecules called neurotransmitters, like acetylcholine, which helps your muscles function properly, is involved with memory, and helps to keep your heart beating.

## Benefits

- **Maintains heart health:** Research shows that when choline intake is optimized, heart disease risk goes down.

- **Can lessen anxiety and affect mental health:** A large study looked at the impact of choline on anxiety levels. People who had lower choline had higher anxiety. More data is needed, but in the meantime, eating a choline-rich diet is a good idea if you struggle with anxiety or other mental health issues.
- **Feeds Your Brain:** Think of choline as food for your brain. It's part of the neurotransmitter (that special messenger molecule) acetylcholine, which impacts memory, mood, and even intelligence. Getting enough choline can boost brain function.

## Side Effects, Warnings, and Precautions

Choline can actually be dangerous in high doses, but this is only a concern if it is obtained through supplements—one more reason why eating your vitamins is so important. Taking high amounts of choline supplements (more than the upper limit of 3,500 milligrams/day for adults) has been linked to side effects like liver damage, low blood pressure, fish odor, throwing up, and excess sweat production.

## Signs of Deficiency

Signs of deficiency can include:

- **Increased risk of problems during pregnancy:** Research shows that women who increase choline during pregnancy may lower the risk of having a baby with a brain or spinal cord birth defect.
- **Nonalcoholic fatty liver disease (NAFLD):** Choline helps to transport fat out of the liver. If there's not enough choline to do its job properly, fat will start to build up in the liver, leading to NAFLD.
- **Low energy:** Since choline is involved in so many key bodily functions, such as muscle movement, DNA synthesis, and even detoxification, inadequate amounts can cause low energy and sluggishness.

## How Much You Need

We still don't know enough about choline to establish a Recommended Daily Allowance. In cases like this, the Institute of Medicine estimates an Adequate Intake (AI), which is the recommended daily intake based on observation and experimentation of healthy groups of people. We do know that the need for choline is affected by various factors, such as genes, activity level, and gender, so the following figures could change in the future.

| AGE | MALE | FEMALE |
|---|---|---|
| 0–6 months | 125mg | 125mg |
| 7–12 months | 150mg | 150mg |
| 1–3 years | 200mg | 200mg |
| 4–8 years | 250mg | 250mg |
| 9–13 years | 375mg | 375mg |
| 14–18 years | 550mg | 400mg |
| 19+ years | 550mg | 425mg |
| Pregnancy | – | 450mg |
| Lactation | – | 550mg |

## Best Way to Consume

Eating a rich variety of foods, particularly protein and some vegetables, is the best way to get choline. Vegans and vegetarians have to be especially conscious of their choline intake, as plant-based products contain much less choline than animal sources. One way to boost your choline intake is to combine eggs with plant-based foods. Two large eggs provide about 300 milligrams of choline, and an adult male needs around 550 milligrams. A great choline-rich meal would be something like a two-egg scramble with shiitake mushrooms and broccoli. You could also throw in some turmeric and olive oil for the anti-inflammatory and additional heart health benefits, plus a handful of greens since they are high in folate and can support your own internal production of choline.

## Natural Food Sources

Since choline was classified only recently, we don't know exactly how much of it exists in a lot of different foods. The following list provides an overview of foods high in choline; however, the list will likely change as more research is done.

| FOOD (SERVING SIZE) | CHOLINE (MG) |
|---|---|
| Beef liver, pan fried (3 ounces) | 356 |
| Egg, hard-boiled (1 large) | 147 |
| Soybeans, roasted (½ cup) | 107 |
| Chicken breast, meat only, roasted (3 ounces) | 72 |
| Beef, ground, 93% lean meat, dry heat (3 ounces) | 72 |
| Codfish, Atlantic, cooked (3 ounces) | 71 |
| Mushrooms, shiitake, cooked (½ cup) | 58 |
| Red potato, baked, flesh and skin (1 large) | 57 |
| Kidney beans, canned, drained (½ cup) | 45 |

| FOOD (SERVING SIZE) | CHOLINE (MG) |
| --- | --- |
| Quinoa, cooked (1 cup) | 43 |
| Brussels sprouts, boiled, drained (½ cup) | 32 |
| Broccoli, chopped, boiled, drained (½ cup) | 31 |
| Cauliflower, boiled (½ cup) | 24 |

## RECIPE

# Egg and Rosemary Scramble *Serves 1*

Eggs are one of the easiest, fastest, and most affordable ways to get a high amount of choline. Rosemary adds a unique, savory twist to this simple recipe.

2 teaspoons extra-virgin olive oil

¼ cup chopped onion

½ cup chopped dandelion greens

¼ cup seeded, chopped orange bell pepper

2 large eggs

1 teaspoon chopped fresh rosemary

2 tablespoons low-fat milk (or milk substitute of your choice)

Pinch salt

Pinch black pepper

**PER SERVING**
*Calories: 276, Fat: 18g, Protein: 15g, Sodium: 469mg, Fiber: 3g, Carbohydrates: 11g, Sugar: 4g, Choline: 305mg*

1 Warm oil over medium heat in a medium cast-iron or nonstick skillet. Add onion and sauté 2–3 minutes, then add greens and bell pepper and sauté another 2–3 minutes.
2 While veggies are cooking, beat eggs in a small bowl with rosemary, milk, salt, and pepper.
3 Add egg mixture to skillet and gently mix with vegetables. Cook until egg mixture cooks all the way through, about 3–4 minutes.
4 Remove to a plate and enjoy!

# Chromium

The ancient Greeks had a word for "color": *chróma*. This is the origin of chromium's name. In nature, chromium is a metal found in many different pigments, such as orange, green, purple, and black. In our bodies, chromium is essential in tiny amounts and is incredibly powerful. A 1960s study looked at hospital patients who were being fed via an IV. They mysteriously developed diabetes symptoms, until it was realized that chromium played a role. They received chromium supplementation, and the diabetes symptoms resolved. For some time now, we've known that chromium is necessary for the body to use insulin and blood sugar properly. It also helps break down and store carbs, fats, and proteins. There's still a lot we do not know about this interesting trace mineral. Read on to learn how to obtain it from your diet.

## Description

Chromium is found in different chemical forms, some of which are toxic, others not edible, and a few that are actually tolerated by the body. Even those forms that are tolerated typically have pretty low absorption rates. The trivalent (3+) form is what humans need and what we'll be referring to here exclusively. Chromium is like an insulin booster. It helps insulin do its job, which is to tell your tissues and cells to use and store the food you eat.

Chromium is found in a wide variety of foods, but most have very small amounts. The amount can vary even in the same types of foods, depending on the soil the food is grown in and how it was processed. Even when you consume foods that have chromium, only tiny amounts of it are absorbed. The more highly processed the food, the less chromium it's likely to have. Interestingly, some other nutrients can boost chromium absorption, and some can have the opposite effect. For example, eating fruits, vegetables, and whole grains can help to increase uptake of chromium in your gut, because they contain vitamin C and niacin, which help with chromium absorption. On the flip side, drinking soda and other sugary drinks, and eating simple carbs (white bread, cakes, muffins, and so on) can actually cause the body to flush out some of its chromium and can eventually even lead to chromium deficiency.

## Role in the Body

- **Insulin enhancer:** Chromium is part of a molecule called chromodulin, which helps insulin do its job properly.

- **Metabolism of macronutrients:** Helps break down carbs, protein, and fats and ensures that they are either used or stored.

## Benefits

- **Helps to keep blood sugar levels stable:** When there is sufficient chromium, you can adequately respond to carbs and sugars from your foods and use or store them, so that your blood sugar remains in balance.
- **May reduce cravings and hunger:** One study showed that a chromium supplement could potentially help reduce cravings and binge-eating episodes. More research is needed, however, to see if these results can be replicated and if this is a benefit from chromium in foods as well.
- **May help with weight management/ weight loss:** This is still a preliminary finding, and more research is needed to determine how chromium affects weight. However, some studies looking at chromium and weight found that there seem to be some beneficial effects.

## Side Effects, Warnings, and Precautions

Interactions between chromium and other nutrients can occur. Iron and chromium compete with each other to be transported in the body. Vitamin C may enhance chromium uptake if the two are consumed together. Diets high in simple sugar increase chromium excretion by urine.

If you are taking chromium supplements, adverse effects can occur if the amount taken exceeds the recommended dose (25–45mcg/day for adults); these effects include headache, diarrhea, fatigue, dizziness, nausea, vomiting, and hives.

Chromium supplements have medication interactions as well, one of the most important being with insulin, so make sure to discuss this and any other supplement you take with your doctor.

## Signs of Deficiency

Deficiency is rare and can occur in people who eat a lot of highly processed foods and sugary drinks, and possibly older adults as they age. There's currently no well-established method for measuring chromium levels in the body, so our knowledge of levels during different life stages is limited. However, it seems that less chromium is either absorbed or more may be excreted as we get older, so ensuring that you get plenty of chromium-containing foods (which is not difficult, because it's found in such a wide variety of sources!) is important.

Signs of deficiency can include:

- Impaired glucose metabolism/progression to diabetes
- Low energy/fatigue
- Increased anxiety

## How Much You Need

There is currently not enough information to establish an RDA for chromium, so the following table lists Adequate Intake (AI) values:

| AGE | MALE | FEMALE |
|---|---|---|
| 0–6 months | 0.2mcg | 0.2mcg |
| 7–12 months | 5.5mcg | 5.5mcg |
| 1–3 years | 11mcg | 11mcg |
| 4–8 years | 15mcg | 15mcg |
| 9–13 years | 25mcg | 21mcg |
| 14–18 years | 35mcg | 24mcg |
| 19–50 years | 35mcg | 25mcg |
| 51+ years | 30mcg | 20mcg |
| Pregnancy | – | 29–30mcg |
| Lactation | – | 44–45mcg |

## Best Way to Consume

There's limited data on how chromium and chromium supplements are absorbed in humans and we also don't have a good method (yet) for testing chromium levels. Some tests of hair, sweat, and blood indicate that chromium levels may decrease with age, so older people may need to consume additional foods that contain it, though much more research is needed in this area to confirm this theory, which is why the AI intake table does not reflect an increase in the recommendation for older adults.

Chromium is a trace mineral, which means you need it in trace (tiny) amounts. Eating a colorful diet with few highly processed foods and a good amount (more than five servings per day) of fruits and vegetables should ensure that you're getting enough. The safety of chromium supplements hasn't been researched in depth, and the quality varies widely, so unless you are unable to consume foods high in chromium, a supplement is likely not warranted.

## Natural Food Sources

| FOOD (SERVING SIZE) | CHROMIUM (MCG) |
|---|---|
| Broccoli, raw, chopped (½ cup) | 11 |
| Potato, mashed (1 cup) | 3 |
| Garlic, dried (1 teaspoon) | 3 |
| Basil, dried (1 teaspoon) | 2 |
| Beef (3 ounces) | 2 |

| FOOD (SERVING SIZE) | CHROMIUM (MCG) |
| --- | --- |
| Whole-wheat bread (2 slices) | 2 |
| Banana, peeled (1 medium) | 1 |
| Green beans, chopped (½ cup) | 1 |
| Black pepper (2 teaspoons) | 0.93 |

## RECIPE

# Colorful Chromium-Rich Chickpea Salad with Broccoli *Serves 2*

In addition to being a great source of chromium and other micronutrients, this recipe also has a good amount of plant-based protein, which will keep you satiated and help you satisfy cravings.

### SALAD

1 cup cooked quinoa

1 cup chopped broccoli florets

½ cup (rinsed and drained, if canned) chickpeas

¼ cup dried cranberries

¼ cup chopped walnuts

### DRESSING

½ tablespoon extra-virgin olive oil

½ tablespoon lemon juice

¼ teaspoon minced garlic

Pinch salt

Pinch black pepper

**PER SERVING**
*Calories: 311, Fat: 15g, Protein: 11g, Sodium: 200mg, Fiber: 8g, Carbohydrates: 36g, Sugar: 4g, Chromium: 14mcg (estimated)*

1  Cook quinoa according to instructions, then remove from pot and set aside.

2  Blanch broccoli florets: Bring a small amount of water to a boil in a small saucepan, then add broccoli and cook 2–3 minutes (just enough so that the broccoli is bright green and tender).

3  In a medium bowl, mix broccoli and quinoa and let cool.

4  Prepare the dressing by whisking together oil, lemon juice, garlic, salt, and pepper in a small bowl. Set aside.

5  Once the quinoa mixture is at room temperature, add chickpeas, cranberries, and walnuts.

6  Add the dressing just before serving.

# Cobalt

Did you know that cobalt is a metal that has been cherished for millennia? It's the source of the bold blue hues in ancient Egyptian stained glass and traditional Chinese ceramics. Today, it's a key component in something we arguably consider even more valuable than art—our electronic devices. Cobalt is one of the essential components of iPhone and Tesla batteries. It's also an essential component of your body. Cobalt is one of the most underrated nutrients. It's sort of like the unsung hero of the mineral world. This mineral is not only essential as an integral part of vitamin $B_{12}$; it's also a powerful nutrient all on its own, as you'll read in this section.

## Description

Cobalt is a mineral that is the thirty-third most common element in the earth's crust. While you only need it in tiny amounts, it plays a big role in your health. There's not a tremendous amount of research on cobalt and how much you need to consume; in fact, there's not even an official Recommended Daily Amount (RDA) for cobalt. However, recent analysis, such as a 2018 article published in *Nutrition*, points to an underappreciation of some of the amazing qualities of cobalt, such as its antioxidant and anti-inflammatory effects. Since many of the foods that contain cobalt are easy to access and are full of other highly beneficial nutrients, cobalt is a mineral you should likely be paying closer attention to.

Cobalt is considered essential for the body because it is a part of vitamin $B_{12}$. Vitamin $B_{12}$ is also known as cobalamin because it depends on cobalt for its synthesis. This conversion usually happens via bacteria that reside in the stomachs of ruminants— this is why the main source of dietary cobalt is through intake of $B_{12}$, and why you get most of it from animal sources.

## Role in the Body

- **Necessary for making red blood cells:** As part of $B_{12}$, cobalt is necessary for making red blood cells in the right amount and proper size.
- **Helps your nervous system to work properly:** Cobalt helps with the formation and repair of nerve ending covers, called myelin.
- **Can replace the action of some minerals:** Cobalt can step in and take the place of some other minerals, like zinc and manganese, when needed.

## Benefits

- **Prevention of anemia:** Lack of $B_{12}$ causes a type of anemia, so cobalt plays a role in preventing this.
- **Adequate functioning of metabolism:** Cobalt is implicated in the production of some enzymes, including thyroxine, one of the thyroid hormones. The thyroid regulates metabolism.
- **Might reduce inflammation:** More research is needed, but cobalt may have the potential to help reduce inflammation in the body, which is a main driver of illness and disease.
- **Aid with potential antioxidant defenses:** This area needs more research, but limited research indicates that cobalt may stimulate certain antioxidant enzymes as well as detoxification enzymes.

## Side Effects, Warnings, and Precautions

Large doses of cobalt can cause toxicity. Some symptoms of severe toxicity include:

- Skin rash
- Overproduction of red blood cells
- Infertility
- Dermatitis
- Panic attacks
- Heart failure

## Signs of Deficiency

A cobalt deficiency usually goes hand-in-hand with lack of $B_{12}$. Signs of deficiency can include:

- Numbness
- Anemia
- Severe fatigue
- Tingling in the hands and feet
- Shortness of breath

## How Much You Need

A safe RDA for cobalt has not yet been determined; however, some sources recommend the following amounts per day, which still need further validation and research but are a potential starting point for evaluating cobalt intake.

| AGE | MALE | FEMALE |
| --- | --- | --- |
| 0–12 months | 0.006mcg | 0.006mcg |
| 1–3 years | 0.006mcg | 0.006mcg |
| 4–8 years | 0.006mcg | 0.006mcg |
| 9–13 years | 10–20mcg | 10–20mcg |
| 14–18 years | 10–20mcg | 10–20mcg |
| 19+ years | 10–20mcg | 10–20mcg |

## Best Way to Consume

Trace amounts of cobalt are found in most foods. Foods high in vitamin $B_{12}$ are the only established sources of cobalt used by the body, though early-stage research seems to indicate that free cobalt (that which is not found in $B_{12}$ and which comes from numerous other sources, such as plants and fish) may play more of a role than previously thought.

## Natural Food Sources

There is very little information on amounts of cobalt in food sources, but here is a list of foods that contain cobalt:

- Whole wheat
- Milk
- Nuts
- Figs
- Green leafy vegetables
- Cabbage
- Shellfish
- Sea vegetables

## RECIPE

# Grain Bowl with Buckwheat  *Serves 2*

Buckwheat is an ancient grain and a true superfood. It is packed with nutrients and has a mild, nutty flavor. This recipe combines healthy ingredients into a flavorful, satisfying meal.

| | | |
|---|---|---|
| 1 cup arugula | 1 tablespoon roasted pine nuts | Pinch salt |
| 1 cup cooked buckwheat | | Pinch black pepper |
| ¼ cup shredded red cabbage | 1 small fig, sliced | 1 tablespoon extra-virgin olive oil |
| ¼ medium avocado, peeled, pitted, and sliced | 2 tablespoons chopped fresh parsley | 1 teaspoon honey |
| 1 ounce feta cheese | ¼ teaspoon red pepper flakes | |

**PER SERVING**
*Calories: 260, Fat: 15g, Protein: 6g, Sodium: 285mg, Fiber: 5g, Carbohydrates: 27g, Sugar: 8g*

1  Add arugula to a medium bowl. Top with buckwheat and cabbage.
2  Add avocado to bowl. Sprinkle with feta, pine nuts, and fig slices.
3  Add parsley, red pepper, salt, and black pepper. Drizzle with oil followed by some honey. Serve.

# Copper

Copper is a trace mineral that you don't hear about too often, though it has many important functions. Without it, you wouldn't be able to create new red blood cells, make collagen, or fight off illness efficiently. As with most nutrients, it's necessary to keep your intake in balance. Too much or too little can have negative effects. Imbalance of this mineral has been linked to Alzheimer's disease. Both deficiency and toxicity are rare and are generally only seen in certain genetic conditions. An interesting fact about copper is that up until 1982, pennies used to be made almost entirely (95 percent) out of copper, but when this mineral became too expensive, pennies cost more to make than their face value. Now, pennies are made mostly out of zinc, with only about 2.5 percent copper. Despite the fact that deficiency is not common, it's still a good idea to incorporate foods that contain some copper into your diet, as they typically come with many other nutrients.

## Description

In early civilizations, copper was prized for its beauty and functionality. In ancient Egypt, copper had many different uses, including in pipes, mirrors, jewelry, obelisks, and decorations on holy temples. Today, it's still used in piping, jewelry, electrical equipment (it's a great conductor of electrical energy), and, of course, in your body. Two of the most important functions of copper in your system are synthesis of red blood cells and energy production. Copper is like the mailman when it comes to picking up iron and delivering it; it's part of a molecule that scoops up iron in the gut and carries it to the tissues in the body, where it's used in the formation of red blood cells. Copper is also an essential player in energy production in every single cell in the body. Copper tends to be concentrated in areas of the body that have extremely high levels of activity, such as the liver, kidneys, heart, brain, skeleton, and muscle.

## Role in the Body

- **Synthesis of red blood cells:** Copper is an integral part of molecules that help to both transport iron and convert it to a form that is usable by the body.
- **Collagen and elastin production:** Copper helps speed up a biochemical reaction that leads to the formation of elastin and collagen in the body, both

of which are needed for healthy skin, joints, and tissues.

- **Immunity:** White blood cells, which surround and destroy invaders inside the body, have been shown to gather copper and use it as a weapon against these intruders. Not enough copper, then, weakens the immune system. Conversely, too much copper is toxic.
- **Helps your body develop melanin:** As part of the enzyme (helper molecule) tyrosinase, copper helps catalyze two different chemical reactions that lead to the production of melanin, the pigment that produces the variation of color In skin, hair, and eyes.
- **Helps create myelin:** Myelin is a protective layer that insulates your nerve cells and helps conduct signals in the body. Copper is needed to form certain types of fats that compose this protective layer.
- **Formation of enzymes:** Enzymes are like little helper molecules that speed up reactions in the body. Copper is necessary for the formation of numerous enzymes. Two examples include cytochrome c oxidase, a key enzyme used in energy production, and superoxide dismutase, a potent antioxidant that needs copper for its formation.
- **Supports thyroid function:** Copper is necessary to help maintain healthy levels of thyroid hormones.

## Benefits

- Prevents anemia
- Aids with proper functioning of the nervous system
- Contributes to vibrant skin and healthy connective tissues
- Helps to build strong, healthy bones
- Leads to fewer infections and less susceptibility to illness
- Has a potential antioxidant function

## Side Effects, Warnings, and Precautions

Too much copper is toxic to your system, so supplements are usually not recommended, especially since you only need tiny (trace) amounts, which you can easily get from foods. There's conflicting data on the links and potential role of copper in Alzheimer's disease. Copper deposits have been found in the brain plaque formations of people with this degenerative condition. However, it's not clear if copper has a role in the formation of these plaques or if it's there to help prevent them. This is an active area of research and debate among brain specialists, and more research is necessary to make solid conclusions.

## Signs of Deficiency

How do you know if you're not getting enough copper? This can be a bit tricky. Signs of copper deficiency can be pretty subtle. Low copper in the body can lead to nonspecific symptoms like fatigue, weakness, depressed immune function, as well as impaired memory and learning problems. Copper is also important in the function of many metabolic processes, including how your body makes energy), how your body makes blood cells (by increasing iron absorption), and how your body maintains its temperature (by affecting your thyroid).

Signs of deficiency can include:

- Fatigue
- Weakness
- Depressed immune function
- Impaired memory and learning problems
- Poor body temperature regulation
- Anemia
- Poor growth and bone formation

## How Much You Need (Amount Per Day)

| AGE | MALE | FEMALE |
|-----|------|--------|
| 0–6 months | 200mcg (AI) | 200mcg (AI) |
| 7–12 months | 220mcg (AI) | 220mcg (AI) |
| 1–3 years | 340mcg | 340mcg |
| 4–8 years | 440mcg | 440mcg |
| 9–13 years | 700mcg | 700mcg |
| 14–18 years | 890mcg | 890mcg |
| 19–69 years | 900mcg | 900mcg |

| AGE | MALE | FEMALE |
|-----|------|--------|
| 70+ years | 900mcg | 900mcg |
| Pregnancy | – | 1,000mcg |
| Lactation | – | 1,300mcg |

## Tolerable Upper Intake Level

| AGE | MALE | FEMALE |
|-----|------|--------|
| 0–6 months | n/a | n/a |
| 7–12 months | n/a | n/a |
| 1–3 years | 1mg | 1mg |
| 4–8 years | 3mg | 3mg |
| 9–13 years | 5mg | 5mg |
| 14–18 years | 8mg | 8mg |
| 19+ years | 10mg | 10mg |
| Pregnancy | – | 8–10mg |
| Lactation | – | 8–10mg |

## Best Way to Consume

The best way to get copper is from food sources. The nutrient zinc competes with copper for absorption in the body. The correct ratio of both of these minerals is essential to avoid potential health issues and side effects, which can include increased inflammation, decreased immunity, and more. This can be done by consuming adequate food sources of both minerals and avoiding any unnecessary supplementation that could throw one or the other out of balance.

## Natural Food Sources

| FOOD (SERVING SIZE) | COPPER (MCG) |
| --- | --- |
| Liver, beef (2½ ounces) | 10,500 |
| Oysters, cooked with moist heat (3½ ounces) | 5,700 |
| Sunflower seeds, dry roasted (¼ cup) | 600 |
| Mushrooms, white, cooked, drained (½ cup) | 390 |
| Almonds, dry roasted (1 ounce) | 310 |
| Soybeans, cooked (½ cup) | 149 |
| Peanuts, dry roasted (1 ounce) | 120 |

## RECIPE

# Low-Carb Asian Rice Bowl *Serves 1*

Bowls are a great way to pack colorful foods into your diet. This twist on an Asian-style bowl uses cauliflower rice to make it lower in carbs but you can always swap in brown or wild rice for extra complex carbs and fiber.

1 teaspoon sesame oil

1 clove garlic, chopped

½ cup white mushrooms

½ cup frozen edamame beans

1 teaspoon chili flakes

1 teaspoon coconut aminos (or low-sodium soy sauce)

1½ cups cooked cauliflower rice

1 teaspoon sesame seeds

**PER SERVING**
*Calories: 208, Fat: 10g, Protein: 14g, Sodium: 145mg, Fiber: 9g, Carbohydrates: 19g, Sugar: 6g, Copper: 520mcg*

1 Heat oil in a medium skillet over medium heat. Add garlic and cook 1 minute.

2 Add mushrooms and cook about 3 minutes or until softened. Add edamame beans and cook for another 1–2 minutes.

3 Add chili flakes and coconut aminos. Stir to combine.

4 Place cauliflower rice in a serving bowl and top with cooked vegetable mixture. Sprinkle with sesame seeds and enjoy!

# Vitamin D

There has been a tremendous amount of interest and research surrounding vitamin D in recent years. Estimates show that approximately one billion people worldwide have low levels of this key nutrient, and the actual number may be much higher. Vitamin D is important and fascinating, playing a role in everything from bone and immunity health to weight and mood. It is not found in very many foods.

## Description

Vitamin D is technically not a vitamin; it is a hormone your body makes when you expose your skin to sunlight. That's incredible! Think about it—your amazing body has the ability to synthesize a key nutrient! The amount of vitamin D your skin can produce depends on many factors such as season, skin pigmentation, and time of day. Ultraviolet sun rays, which are required to produce vitamin D naturally, are not strong enough in higher latitudes from October to March. If you live in the northern latitudes, you might not be getting enough vitamin D during these months. People with darker skin make less vitamin D, and deficiency levels are much higher among African Americans. Although some foods have a little naturally occurring vitamin D, foods cannot provide enough of this vitamin. So, fortified foods are the best dietary sources.

Your body also manufactures vitamin D from cholesterol through a process triggered by the action of sunlight on skin, hence its nickname, "the sunshine vitamin." Yet many people do not make enough vitamin D from the sun, for a number of reasons—we generally spend less time in the sun than we used to, and we wear sunscreen or cover up when we do.

## Role in the Body

- Helps body absorb calcium
- Regulates immune response

Vitamin D's main role is to help absorb calcium and strengthen bones. Additionally, vitamin D might be protective against cancers because it plays a role in cell differentiation and proliferation. The vitamin D receptor is expressed by many immune cells. Vitamin D acts to regulate the immune response. Some research suggests that it might be protective against several autoimmune conditions such as multiple sclerosis or type 1 diabetes.

## Benefits

- Maintains strong bones
- May improve depression
- May regulate appetite and promote weight loss

Vitamin D helps the body absorb calcium and phosphorus, which helps maintain strong bones. Some research has shown that optimizing vitamin D levels can help improve symptoms of depression. A 2013 study asserts that people taking vitamin D and calcium supplements had an easier time losing weight than those who did not. It was thought that the combination of these nutrients may aid in regulating appetite.

## Side Effects, Warnings, and Precautions

Taking megadoses of vitamin D (around 60,000 international units) will cause toxicity after a few months. The main side effect of vitamin D toxicity is buildup of calcium in the blood (hypercalcemia), which can cause decreased kidney function, nausea, vomiting, and weakness. In the longer term, hypercalcemia results in kidney failure, cardiovascular system failure, and calcification of soft tissues. This is a very rare condition, and most supplements do not have such high amounts, so it's unlikely you need to be concerned about toxicity or getting too much vitamin D.

## Signs of Deficiency

Vitamin D deficiency can decrease the amount of calcium absorbed, so osteoporosis is a big risk factor among those deficient in vitamin D. Signs of mild deficiency include:

- Fatigue
- Low immunity
- Bone pain
- Weakness
- Poor wound healing

## How Much You Need

Different age groups require different amounts of vitamin D. Following are the most recent, updated reference RDA ranges.

It's a good idea to meet with a dietitian to review how much vitamin D you are getting through your diet and lifestyle so you can select the right dose when supplementing.

| Infants 0–12 months | 400 IU (international units)/10mcg (AI) |
| Children 1–18 years | 600 IU/15mcg |
| Adults | 600–1,000 IU/15mcg |
| Adults 70+ years | 800–1,000 IU/20mcg |

## Tolerable Upper Level

| Infants 0–6 months | 1,000 IU (international units)/25mcg |
|---|---|
| Infants 7–12 months | 1,500 IU/38mcg |
| Children 1–3 years | 2,500 IU/63mcg |
| Children 4–8 years | 3,000 IU/75mcg |
| Over 9 years old | 4,000 IU/100mcg |

## Best Way to Consume

- Take supplements of at least 600 IU per day
- Take supplements with food for best absorption
- Take supplements with a healthy fat source to maximize absorption

Vitamin D is best consumed from supplements at doses of at least 600 IU per day. It helps you to absorb calcium and phosphorus, both of which are needed for bone strength. Because vitamin D is fat-soluble, it is best absorbed when taken with food. Adding a healthy source of fat (such as seafood, avocado, or nuts) will further improve vitamin D absorption.

## Natural Food Sources

Dietary sources of vitamin D are limited. The best way to get vitamin D is through supplementation, though a little bit of sun exposure will also help to raise levels. Some vitamin D can be found in dairy products, seafood, and other fortified foods. Some foods that contain vitamin D include:

- Salmon
- Sardines
- Egg yolk
- Shrimp
- Mushrooms
- Milk (fortified)
- Cereal (fortified)
- Yogurt (fortified)
- Orange juice (fortified)

# Superfood Sardine Salad  *Serves 2*

Sardines are one of the best fish you can eat. They are full of the uber-healthy omega-3 fatty acids DHA and EPA, which promote brain health, heart health, and a host of other benefits. Sardines tend to be lower in mercury than many other fish and high in protein. Make sure you are selecting sustainably sourced sardines when you purchase them. You can do this by looking at the Seafood Watch list of fish and also buying fish that have the MSC (Marine Stewardship Council) label. This creative dish is easy to make and can turn even someone who thinks they don't like sardines into a fan. You can substitute the sardines with tuna, salmon, or any other canned fish if you want, but you should really try the sardines!

1 (6-ounce) can sardines in water

1 large tomato, chopped

1 medium stalk celery, chopped

1 small cucumber, chopped

¼ medium head cabbage, purple or green, shredded

1 tablespoon extra-virgin olive oil

1 tablespoon balsamic vinegar

Pinch sea salt

Pinch black pepper

1 teaspoon ground mustard

⅛ teaspoon turmeric

**PER SERVING**

*Calories: 273, Fat: 14g, Protein: 20g, Sodium: 503mg, Fiber: 5g, Carbohydrates: 18g, Sugar: 10g, Vitamin D: 87mcg/3,480IU*

1  Drain sardines, place into a large mixing bowl.

2  Add the rest of the ingredients and toss well to combine. Taste and adjust salt and pepper as needed. Enjoy!

# Vitamin E

The benefits of vitamin E make it sound like a wonder drug: repairing the skin, slowing down aging, powerful antioxidant properties, possible help with Alzheimer's, protecting vision, and much more. A fascinating nutrient, vitamin E is actually a group of eight different compounds. The most well known and well studied by far is alpha-tocopherol, which boosts immunity and helps keep blood clots from forming. Some of the other compounds—especially tocotrienols, which may help prevent free radical damage to the gastrointestinal system among other benefits—are starting to get more attention for their health potential. Let's dive in to find out more about this outstanding nutrient, where to get it, and what to watch out for.

## Description

Part of the fat-soluble family of vitamins, vitamin E is found in a variety of foods including nuts, seeds, and oils, as well as in some fruits and vegetables (in smaller amounts). A potent vitamin, it's important for skin and hair health, vision, immune system, and reproduction. There has been quite a bit of interesting research on the effects of vitamin E on various conditions such as heart disease, cancers, and brain health. Although vitamin E supplements are popular, most people don't need them and will reap the most benefit from increasing their intake of healthful foods that are high in the vitamin.

The eight different compounds of vitamin E are split into four tocopherol forms and four tocotrienol forms. We know that the main tocopherol, alpha-tocopherol, is present in the highest amounts in your blood and has the most bioactive effects. Because it is the best absorbed, alpha-tocopherol is the most well-known form and so much of the traditional research has focused on it. More recent research has focused on some of the other forms, with evidence emerging that tocotrienol forms, while rarer and harder to get from food sources, may also have valuable effects, such as potent antioxidant activity, especially in the gut.

## Role in the Body

- **Functions as an antioxidant:** This is the main benefit of vitamin E. It protects body tissues and organs from damage by free radicals (compounds that damage cells when not neutralized by antioxidants) and plays a role in keeping cholesterol levels in check and thus reducing risk of heart disease and stroke.

- **Boosts immune system:** Protects the body against viruses and bacteria by helping to ensure that T-cells—which play a big role in cell immunity—divide properly so they can function in the right way.
- **Anti-inflammatory:** Vitamin E has powerful anti-inflammatory activities especially related to heart health and arteries.
- **Signal transmission between cells:** Vitamin E controls some signal transmission pathways and proteins, especially in the liver and gastrointestinal tract.
- **Tocotrienols:** There's not a lot of research on tocotrienols, but we do know they play a valuable role, such as reduction of inflammation, helping your brain stay healthy, and possibly protecting you from Alzheimer's and Parkinson's diseases.

## Benefits

- **Protects against cancer:** Since vitamin E has strong antioxidant properties and can reduce the damage from free radicals, it protects the body against cancer.
- **Promotes skin regeneration and wound healing:** Vitamin E protects the skin from UV light and can help to heal dark spots, wrinkles, and wounds.
- **Can help to prevent heart disease:** Vitamin E prevents the buildup of fatty plaque on artery walls, which lowers the risk of heart disease.
- **Promotes eye health:** Vitamin E protects your eyes from age-related diseases.
- **Can help with PMS symptoms:** Vitamin E possibly reduces painful cramps, cravings, and depression in some women.

## Side Effects, Warnings, and Precautions

While getting vitamin E from foods is very safe, taking supplemental doses of vitamin E in high amounts can actually have the opposite effects from what is desired. Although research on supplemental vitamin E is mixed, it does indicate that high doses of vitamin E can increase the risk of bleeding and stroke, can reduce the effects of some medications like blood thinners, and can also reduce the effectiveness of vitamin K. Make sure you discuss any supplements you take with your doctor and dietitian before starting them, especially if you have any heart conditions or are taking other medications.

## Signs of Deficiency

Deficiency can occur in people who have issues with fat absorption, including individuals who have had recent bariatric (weight loss) surgeries, people with cystic fibrosis, and babies who are born early or at a very low birth weight. Signs of deficiency include:

- **Blunted immune system response:** Your body may not be as effective in responding to illness and fighting off infections if your vitamin E intake isn't optimal.
- **Nerve and muscle impairment:** Since vitamin E is important for signal transmission between cells and communication, lack of it could lead to damage and impairment.
- **Vision impairment and damage.** Vitamin E is necessary for the retina of the eye to function properly, and low levels can cause retinal damage.

## How Much You Need

The RDA for vitamin E is as follows (note that the data in the following table refers only to alpha-tocopherol, since this is the only form of vitamin E that has been studied in depth). Also, effective January 1, 2021, vitamin E will be listed in milligrams rather than international units, per new labeling regulations. The following table uses milligrams to avoid any confusion.

| AGE | MALE | FEMALE |
| --- | --- | --- |
| 0–6 months | 4mg (AI not RDA)* | 4mg (AI not RDA)* |
| 7–12 months | 5mg (AI not RDA)* | 5mg (AI not RDA)* |
| 1–3 years | 6mg | 6mg |
| 4–8 years | 7mg | 7mg |
| 9–13 years | 11mg | 11mg |
| 14+ years | 15mg | 15mg |
| Pregnancy | – | 15mg |
| Lactation | – | 19mg |

* Adequate Intake amounts were developed for infants because there isn't sufficient evidence for a Recommended Daily Allowance (RDA).

## Best Way to Consume

Consuming vitamin E from foods is preferable to getting it from supplements whenever possible. In some cases, such as with premature infants and people with absorption disorders, supplements are necessary. Vitamin E is absorbed at higher rates from food sources (it is more bioavailable) and comes with a host of other benefits such as all the other vitamins, minerals, and fiber when consumed from whole foods. You also don't run the risk of overconsuming it when getting it from food sources, as is the case with most vitamins and nutrients. It's also important to remember that vitamin E is destroyed by high heat, so cooking with oils at a high temperature, such as frying, will reduce or eliminate the vitamin E in the oil.

## Natural Food Sources

| FOOD (SERVING SIZE) | VITAMIN E (MG) |
| --- | --- |
| Wheatgerm oil (1 tablespoon) | 20.3 |
| Sunflower seeds, dry roasted (2 tablespoons) | 7.4 |
| Almonds, dry roasted (2 tablespoons) | 6.8 |
| Hazelnuts, dry roasted (2 tablespoons) | 4.3 |
| Pine nuts (¼ cup) | 3 |
| Peanut butter (2 tablespoons) | 2.9 |
| Egg, cooked (2 large) | 2.3 |
| Sardines, canned with oil, drained (⅓ cup) | 2 |
| Spinach, boiled (½ cup) | 1.9 |
| Turnip greens, cooked (½ cup) | 1.4 |
| Broccoli, chopped, boiled, drained (½ cup) | 1.1 |
| Kiwifruit (1 medium) | 1.1 |
| Avocado (¼ medium) | 0.8 |

## Foods High in Tocotrienols

More research is needed to determine specific amounts for these foods, but if you want to get more tocotrienols, the lesser known forms of vitamin E that seem to have potent antioxidant effects in your diet, here are some foods to incorporate.

- Flaxseed
- Annatto seeds
- Palm fruit
- Rice bran
- Oats
- Pumpkin seeds
- Barley
- Rye
- Sunflower seeds

## RECIPE

# Skin Glow Smoothie *Serves 1*

This smoothie is packed with vitamin E, which helps your skin stay healthy. Starting your day with this nutrient-packed meal will make you feel glorious!

| | | |
|---|---|---|
| 1 cup unsweetened almond milk | ½ cup frozen nectarine chunks | 1 tablespoon almond butter |
| 1 medium kiwifruit, peeled | ½ medium frozen banana, peeled | 2 teaspoons wheat germ |
| | ½ cup spinach | Ice cubes, as needed |

**PER SERVING**
*Calories: 273, Fat: 12g, Protein: 8g, Sodium: 194mg, Fiber: 8g, Carbohydrates: 39g, Sugar: 20g, Vitamin E (alpha-tocopherol): 1,011mg*

Add all ingredients to a blender and mix well. Enjoy immediately.

# Fiber

Did you know there are actually several types of fiber, each of which has a wide variety of benefits in your body? Foods that contain fiber have varying amounts of it and usually a combination of some of these different types. You don't really need to think about the specific type when you're choosing fibrous foods; what's most important is that you get enough overall fiber. If you are getting enough fiber, then you'll likely be getting a mix of the different varieties of this awesome nutrient.

## Description

Fiber is the only nutrient that isn't fully digested or absorbed, which means it helps with appetite, weight loss, cholesterol levels, and so much more.

There are two main classes of fibers: soluble and insoluble. Soluble fibers dissolve in water and become gummy-like. These kinds of fibers help with digestion, lower cholesterol levels, and help to slow down increases in blood sugar. Insoluble fibers don't dissolve in water, but they do retain water in the colon and add bulk to the stools. Fiber has a strong detoxifying effect because it actually binds to wastes and toxins and helps to remove them from your system quickly and efficiently.

Some of the main types of fiber are as follows:

| FIBER TYPE (S = SOLUBLE AND I = INSOLUBLE) | FUNCTION |
| --- | --- |
| Betaglucan (s) | Has been shown to lower "bad'" cholesterol, thus being heart protective |
| Inulin (s) (not to be confused with insulin) | Fermentable fiber, also acts as a prebiotic |
| Lignin (i) | Prevents constipation, increases the rate at which wastes are removed |
| Cellulose (i) | Aids digestion, acts like a natural "broom" |
| Hemicellulose (i) (s) | Slows stomach emptying, helping with feelings of fullness |
| Gums (s) | Lower cholesterol |
| Pectins (s) | Lower blood sugar, are fermentable |
| Mucilages (s) | Reduce absorption of fats and cholesterol |

## Role in the Body

- **Weight management:** Research has repeatedly shown that a high-fiber diet is correlated with a lower weight.
- **Detoxification and waste elimination:** Insoluble fiber binds to waste products and toxins, sweeping them out of the body and acting like a detox mechanism.
- **Blood sugar regulation:** Eating more fiber, especially soluble fiber, has been shown to slow down the rise of blood sugar levels after a meal.
- **Satiety/fullness:** Fiber-full meals have more "roughage," feel more filling, and take more time to eat, helping you to feel more satisfied with fewer calories.
- **Prebiotic function:** Many fibers act as prebiotics, providing a food source for the good gut bacteria in your digestive tract.
- **Production of short-chain fatty acids:** Some fermentable fibers are used by bacteria in your gut to make short-chain fatty acids, which help increase absorption of some vitamins and minerals, strengthen the immune system, and even give you an energy boost.
- **Gut health:** Fiber is essential for a healthy digestive tract and regular bowel movements. Fermentable fibers (found in foods like beans and legumes) provide the perfect environment for colonies of beneficial bacteria to thrive, thus boosting immunity and even reducing issues from food sensitivities and intolerances.
- **Heart health:** Some fibers help to lower the levels of "bad" cholesterol.
- **Immunity:** Fiber can suppress growth of harmful bacteria as well as lower inflammation.

## Benefits

- Maintenance of a healthy weight and weight loss
- Natural detoxifier
- Stronger immune system
- Lower blood sugar levels
- Healthy gut function
- Lower risk of heart disease
- Improved cholesterol levels
- Reduced risk of certain cancers (especially colon cancer) and infections
- Reduced risk of hemorrhoids (painful, swollen veins near the anus) due to less straining and softer stools
- May help to reduce blood pressure
- Improved intestinal pH levels
- Better absorption of some key vitamins and minerals

## Side Effects, Warnings, and Precautions

Increasing fiber suddenly can cause intestinal upset and symptoms like bloating, gas, and diarrhea. This is temporary, and your body should adjust over one to four weeks to the increased amount. Because of this, you should introduce more fiber slowly, increasing the amount a little bit each day over a period of months.

People who follow a low-FODMAP (fermentable oligosaccharides, disaccharides, monosaccharides, and polyols) diet usually need to be cautious about how much fiber they eat. If this is your situation, you should meet with a dietitian who specializes in digestive health to help you.

## Signs of Deficiency

Most people in the US are deficient in fiber because we typically under consume high fiber foods, which include vegetables, legumes, and whole grains. People with gastrointestinal problems such as irritable bowel syndrome (IBS), who have a hard time eating enough fiber, could also be low in this nutrient. Signs of deficiency can include:

- Fatigue/weakness
- Constipation/irregular bowel movements
- Digestive discomfort
- Gut dysbiosis/imbalance
- Increased susceptibility to illness and infection

## How Much You Need

There is no tolerable upper limit set for fiber, but anything above 60 grams or so can start to interfere with the absorption of vitamins, minerals, and other beneficial compounds, as well as cause GI upset. It's hard to get this amount from foods, but it's possible by taking too many fiber supplements.

The AI for fiber is:

| AGE | MALE | FEMALE |
| --- | --- | --- |
| 0–12 months | – | – |
| 1–3 years | 19g | 19g |
| 4–8 years | 25g | 25g |
| 9–13 years | 31g | 26g |
| 14–18 years | 38g | 26g |
| 19–50 years | 38g | 25g |
| 51+ years | 30g | 21g |
| Pregnancy | – | 28g |
| Lactation | – | 29g |

## Best Way to Consume

Fiber is found in foods that are not highly processed, so fruits and vegetables in their natural packaging (skin!) are an awesome source, leafy greens are excellent, and legumes such as beans and lentils are the top source of fiber-rich foods (but not processed ones like refried beans). Seeds and nuts have fiber as well, and all whole grains contain fiber.

You should get *all* of your fiber from food as opposed to supplements, unless there's a medical condition that prevents you from being able to eat enough fiber.

## Natural Food Sources

| FOOD (SERVING SIZE) | FIBER | SOLUBLE | INSOLUBLE |
|---|---|---|---|
| Lentils, cooked (1 cup) | 15.6g | 6.73g | 8.87g |
| Black beans (1 cup) | 15g | 5.4g | 9.6g |
| Chickpeas, canned, drained (1 cup) | 12g | 3.87g | 9.87g |
| Oats, dry (1¼ cups) | 10g | 4.2g | 5.8g |
| Corn bran (1 cup) | 7.9g | 0.24g | 7.66g |
| Collardgreens, frozen (1 cup) | 4.8g | 2.39g | 2.41g |
| Avocado, medium (1 whole) | 3.5g | 1.95g | 1.55g |
| Brown rice, cooked (1 cup) | 3.5g | 0.39g | 3.11g |
| Hazelnuts (¼ cup) | 3.3g | 1.1g | 2.2g |
| Nectarine (1 medium) | 2.4g | 1.4g | 1.0g |
| Apricots (3 whole) | 2.1g | 1.4g | 0.70g |
| Grapefruit (½ medium) | 1.4g | 1.05g | 0.35g |

# Digestion-Boosting Rainbow Bowl *Serves 1*

This recipe has 35 grams of carbs and 9 grams of fiber, which is about 50 percent or more of your daily fiber goal amount and a really healthy amount of overall carbs—enough to give you plenty of energy and keep you full without spiking your blood sugar.

## SALAD

½ cup chopped Swiss chard

½ cup chopped baby kale

¼ cup cooked lentils

¼ cup riced cauliflower

¼ cup cooked brown rice

¼ cup shredded purple cabbage

1 tablespoon roasted chickpeas

3 cherry tomatoes, halved

## DRESSING

Juice of ½ medium lemon

3 tablespoons water, or more as needed

1 tablespoon creamy tahini

¼ teaspoon garlic powder

1 tablespoon extra-virgin olive oil

Pinch salt

Pinch black pepper

**PER SERVING**
*Calories: 358, Fat: 21g, Protein: 11g, Sodium: 373mg, Fiber: 9g, Carbohydrates: 35g, Sugar: 5g*

1 Assemble all salad ingredients in a medium bowl.

2 In a small bowl, mix the dressing ingredients until smooth. Add more water if needed to reach desired consistency.

3 Drizzle the salad with tahini dressing and enjoy!

# Fluoride

Many vitamins, minerals, and nutritive substances are helpful in small doses, but they can be harmful in large quantities. For example, a little bit of sun is good for you, but too much sun can cause sunburn and put you at risk for skin cancer. We know that fluoride is one of the trace minerals your body uses to maintain healthy, cavity-free teeth. However, fluoride use is a controversial topic, as concerns have been raised about potential harm from getting too much. While we know some of its benefits, it's still not entirely clear if fluoride is truly essential to health. This entry will look at fluoride, the current recommendations regarding its intake, and why it's been so controversial.

## Description

Almost all the fluoride you get in your diet comes from water. Not all water is fluoridated (that is, has fluoride added to it), so the amount that people consume worldwide varies. About 75 percent of fluoride intake in the US comes from water, soft drinks, and juice. More than 300 million people in countries such as Australia, Canada, Malaysia, and the US receive artificially fluoridated water. Countries that have naturally occurring fluoridation include China, Gabon, and Sweden. Many European countries fluoridate salt and milk instead of water. There are different opinions about the benefits of water fluoridation and whether it is healthy or not. Some studies show that water fluoridation helps with dental health but other studies show that topical contact with teeth (just through toothpaste, for example) is enough to get the benefits and there is no need to consume it orally. In 2015, the US Department of Health & Human Services revised its fluoride recommended amount to 0.7 parts per million (ppm) down from 0.7–1.2 previously. This was done to prevent a cosmetic defect called fluorosis, or a discoloration of the teeth, which happens when consuming too much fluoride.

There is plenty of controversy around fluoride. Numerous concerns have been raised about possible neurotoxic effects, especially on the developing brains of children, from additional fluoride. More than fifty studies show that fluoride negatively affects learning and memory in rats and mice. These findings are concerning, but humans typically do not get extremely high doses of fluoride. Also, we metabolize substances differently than rats or mice, so we have to be cautious in how we interpret and apply such findings.

## Role in the Body

- Strengthens tooth enamel
- Prevents cavities
- May strengthen bones

## Benefits

- Fluoridation has been shown to prevent tooth decay and reduce cavities.
- It may help to prevent osteoporosis by strengthening bones.

## Side Effects, Warnings, and Precautions

The US began adding fluoride to the water supply in 1945. In recent years, there has been concern that too much fluoride can cause increased risks of birth defects, cancer, heart disease, liver disease, Alzheimer's disease, and more. However, there is no scientific evidence to support these concerns. Almost any substance, even most vitamins and minerals, will have toxic effects in extremely high doses. The same is true for fluoride. Very high intakes of fluoride can have toxic effects, such as damage to the brain, reduced function of the thyroid gland, and an increased risk for bone fractures and bone cancer. Quantities that are well above the recommended amounts would be required to see these effects, and this is very rare and unlikely without accidental overdose. Based on the available evidence, the current level in our water supply seems to be safe.

The current position of the Academy of Nutrition and Dietetics on fluoride states, "It is the position of the Academy of Nutrition and Dietetics to support optimal systemic and topical fluoride as an important public health measure to promote oral health and overall health throughout life."

## Signs of Deficiency

Signs of deficiency can include:

- Cavities (dental caries)
- Weaker teeth and/or tooth enamel

## How Much You Need

The official recommendations for fluoride were updated in 1997. There was not enough information to set a Recommended Daily Allowance (RDA), so instead, Adequate Intake (AI) levels were established based on the minimum levels that have been shown to decrease cavities without the unwanted side effect of discoloration.

| AGE | MALE | FEMALE |
| --- | --- | --- |
| 0–6 months | 0.01mg | 0.01mg |
| 7–12 months | 0.5mg | 0.5mg |
| 1–3 years | 0.7mg | 0.7mg |
| 4–8 years | 1mg | 1mg |
| 9–13 years | 2mg | 2mg |
| 14–18 years | 3mg | 3mg |

| AGE | MALE | FEMALE |
| --- | --- | --- |
| 19+ years | 4mg | 3mg |
| Pregnancy | – | 3mg |
| Lactation | – | 3mg |

| AGE | MALE | FEMALE |
| --- | --- | --- |
| 19+ years | 10mg | 10mg |
| Pregnancy | – | 10mg |
| Lactation | – | 10mg |

## Upper Level of Intake (Amount Per Day)

| AGE | MALE | FEMALE |
| --- | --- | --- |
| 0–6 months | 0.7mg | 0.7mg |
| 7–12 months | 0.9mg | 0.9mg |
| 1–3 years | 1.3mg | 1.3mg |
| 4–8 years | 2.2mg | 2.2mg |
| 9–13 years | 10mg | 10mg |
| 14–18 years | 10mg | 10mg |

## Best Way to Consume

The majority of the fluoride intake in the US comes from fluoridated water, and most people get enough. Even if you don't drink fluoridated water, it should be sufficient to brush your teeth with toothpaste containing fluoride to obtain the enamel and cavity-fighting benefits.

## Natural Food Sources

The following estimate is dependent on the soil or water content of fluoride where the food is grown.

| FOOD (SERVING SIZE) | FLUORIDE (MG) |
| --- | --- |
| Drinking water, tap (4 cups) | 0.7–1.2 |
| Crab, canned, drained (3½ ounces) | 0.21 |
| Rice, brown, cooked (3½ ounces) | 0.04 |
| Fish, canned, drained, cooked (3½ ounces) | 0.02 |
| Chicken, cooked (3½ ounces) | 0.015 |
| Black tea (4 cups) | 1–5 |
| Carrots, sliced (4 cups) | 0.03 |
| Strawberries, sliced (4 cups) | 0.04 |

# Iodine

Iodine is essential for proper functioning of your thyroid, a tiny, butterfly-shaped organ at the base of your neck. The thyroid is also where most of the iodine in your body is stored. Iodine deficiency is quite common worldwide and has devastating effects. Deficiency in the US greatly declined after salt became fortified with iodine; however, iodized salt is not mandatory in the US, and some research, such as a 2015 article in the journal *Nutrients*, estimates that only about half the population consumes it. In fact, intake of iodine in the West in general has actually *decreased* in recent decades, for numerous reasons, such as the way food is processed and depletion of the soil. Pregnant women are most at risk for inadequate intake, since iodine needs increase to meet those of the growing baby.

## Description

Iodine is like a control lever for critical hormone production that directly affects key processes like your metabolism. If there's too little or too much iodine in the body, it throws the thyroid out of whack and can cause symptoms like fatigue, weight gain, and other thyroid problems. Your thyroid gland makes hormones called T3 and T4, which have iodine as a key component. A condition called goiter—enlargement of the thyroid gland, which is visible as a swollen lump in the neck—is the result of lack of iodine over time. Goiter occurs because the thyroid actually grows larger in an attempt to gather more iodine from circulating levels in the body.

A lot of iodine comes from the ocean, so areas closer to the coast tend to have more iodine in their soil and thus their food, which absorbs some of the iodine from the soil. If you don't live close to the ocean, you may need to pay attention to your iodine intake to make sure you are getting enough.

## Role in the Body

- **Control of metabolism:** The thyroid gland needs iodine to produce thyroid hormones, which control and balance metabolism in the body.
- **Creation of enzymes:** Iodine is one of the components required for the formation of enzymes needed to synthesize thyroid hormones.
- **Strengthening of immune system:** It's been shown that iodine acts as an antioxidant, removing harmful free radicals in the body, and thereby reducing the risk of cancer and other chronic diseases.

- **Brain development in babies:** It is crucial for babies to take in enough iodine to reach the required amount of thyroid hormone to be released and utilized for growth at normal rate.

## Benefits

- **Promotes healthy weight:** Iodine is needed for production of thyroid hormones, which control the speed of metabolism and help to maintain a healthy weight.
- **Contributes to healthy hair and nails:** Having the right amount of iodine helps ensure that hair and nail cells regenerate efficiently.
- **Improves energy and stamina:** Thyroid hormones play an important role in providing energy for the body to function optimally.
- **Boosts immunity:** Iodine reduces the risk of disease by boosting the immune system.
- **Detoxifies:** Iodine has antioxidant characteristics and can remove harmful free radicals in the body.

## Side Effects, Warnings, and Precautions

Too much iodine can cause similar symptoms as iodine deficiency. These include:

- Nausea, vomiting, and diarrhea
- Goiter and inflammation of the thyroid gland

Iodine poisoning is rare; however, if it is consumed in amounts far above the upper limit (multiple grams or more), it can cause acute poisoning with symptoms such as burning of the mouth, throat, and stomach, as well as diarrhea and vomiting.

## Signs of Deficiency

Signs of deficiency can include:

- Feeling cold
- Brittle hair
- Fatigue, weakness
- Swelling of the neck/goiter

## How Much You Need (RDA)

| AGE | MALE | FEMALE |
| --- | --- | --- |
| 0–6 months | 110mcg (AI) | 110mcg (AI) |
| 7–12 months | 130mcg (AI) | 130mcg (AI) |
| 1–3 years | 90mcg | 90mcg |
| 4–8 years | 90mcg | 90mcg |

| AGE | MALE | FEMALE |
|---|---|---|
| 9–13 years | 120mcg | 120mcg |
| 14–18 years | 150mcg | 150mcg |
| 19+ years | 150mcg | 150mcg |
| Pregnancy | – | 220mcg |
| Lactation | – | 290mcg |

## Tolerable Upper Intake Levels for Iodine (Amount Per Day)

| AGE | MALE | FEMALE |
|---|---|---|
| 0–12 months | Not established | Not established |
| 1–3 years | 200mcg | 200mcg |
| 4–8 years | 300mcg | 300mcg |
| 9–13 years | 600mcg | 600mcg |
| 14–18 years | 900mcg | 900mcg |
| 19+ years | 1,100mcg | 1,100mcg |
| Pregnancy | – | 1,100mcg |
| Lactation | – | 1,100mcg |

According to the National Health and Nutrition Examination Survey, about one third of pregnant women are at least mildly deficient in iodine. This is a critical issue, because the growing baby relies on the mother's iodine stores for proper development of the brain. Women who don't consume dairy, seafood, or sea vegetables might have to take an iodine supplement (if it is not already included in their prenatal) to ensure that their and their babies' needs are met.

### Best Way to Consume

There aren't too many foods that contain iodine, so it requires some planning and conscious effort to make sure you are getting enough. It's well worth the effort, though, for all the benefits that iodine provides. Once consumed, iodine is absorbed quickly in the body, and excess is flushed out in the urine.

Some foods contain compounds called goitrogens—these are elements that can block the thyroid from absorbing iodine. They include some vegetables like cabbage, turnips, cassava, broccoli, collard greens, bok choy, Brussels sprouts, cauliflower, kale, spinach, and mustard greens. There is no need to decrease your intake of these vegetables unless you are already low in iodine.

Sea vegetables are an excellent, natural source of iodine. If you don't already eat things like seaweed, kelp, or kombu (the main ingredient in miso soup), try incorporating them into your diet.

Iodized salt is another important source of iodine; try to use this at home when cooking.

If you're not able to meet your iodine needs through your diet, there are a number of different supplements with varying effects and absorption rates. Discuss this with your doctor and dietitian to determine the amount and type that is best for you.

## Natural Food Sources

| FOOD (SERVING SIZE) | IODINE (MCG) |
| --- | --- |
| Seaweed (1 sheet) | 16–2,984<br>(depends on the sourcing; for example, seaweed from Japan tends to have much more iodine than other parts of the world) |
| Sea vegetables (1 tablespoon)<br>(for example, kelp, kombu, arame, wakame, and dulse) | 750 |
| Scallops, steamed (4 ounces) | 135 |
| Cod, baked (3½ ounces) | 115 |
| Yogurt, plain, low-fat (1 cup) | 75 |
| Sardines, canned, drained (4.3 ounces) | 35 |
| Shrimp (3 ounces) | 35 |
| Salmon (4 ounces) | 32 |
| Egg (1 large) | 24 |
| Prunes, dried (5) | 13 |
| Lima beans, boiled (½ cup) | 8 |
| Spinach (1 cup) | 3.60 |

# Homemade Ramen Soup with Kelp Noodles *Serves 2*

Ramen soup is the ultimate comfort food! Make it healthier with kelp noodles and a veggie stock. This low-calorie dish is warm and satisfying.

---

2 cups low-sodium vegetable or mushroom stock

1 teaspoon sesame oil

1 tablespoon minced fresh ginger

½ teaspoon red pepper flakes

1 clove garlic, minced

1 cup sliced mushrooms

1 small head bok choy, chopped

6 ounces kelp noodles

1 sheet nori, sliced lengthwise, for garnish

1 bunch scallions, sliced, for garnish

½ teaspoon soy sauce

---

**PER SERVING**

*Calories: 112, Fat: 3g, Protein: 9g, Sodium: 542mg, Fiber: 7g, Carbohydrates: 20g, Sugar: 10g*

1 Pour vegetable or mushroom stock into a large stockpot. Add sesame oil, ginger, red pepper flakes, and garlic. Bring to a boil, then reduce heat and let simmer 10 minutes.

2 Add mushrooms and bok choy and cook 5 minutes.

3 Add kelp noodles and stir to combine.

4 Garnish with nori, scallions, and soy sauce, and serve.

# Iron

One of the most crucial minerals in your body, iron is essential to keeping you healthy and energized. It has many valuable roles, but one of the most interesting and important is its ability to carry oxygen throughout the body and to every cell. Aside from ferrying oxygen everywhere inside the body, iron is also a key nutrient for brain and body development. Children need the right amount to focus in school and learn properly. But there is a downside to iron: In large amounts it can be toxic. Read on for some amazing facts about iron and how to optimize it and your health.

## Description

Iron is so important that your body evolved to obtain and absorb it in multiple forms: heme and nonheme. Your body can absorb iron from *both* plant (nonheme) and animal (heme) sources. Heme iron is easier to absorb, while nonheme, which comes from things like dark leafy greens and beans, needs a helper. That helper is vitamin C, which boosts the absorption of plant-sourced iron.

Keeping iron at optimal levels is critical, because both too little and too much iron can be harmful. When you have too little iron, you can develop a condition called iron deficiency anemia, which can lead to feeling exhausted, a weakened immune system, risks during pregnancy, and more. Too much iron is also not good. Even though it's an essential mineral, iron is also an oxidant, which means it causes tissue damage and can even increase the risk of certain chronic diseases if overconsumed.

## Role in the Body

- **Production of red blood cells:** Iron helps create red blood cells. Red blood cells turn over every four months or so, and some of the iron inside them is recycled and used again by the body.
- **Carries oxygen to all organ systems, cells, and muscles:** This is the main role of iron in the body and is fundamental to good health and functioning.
- **Necessary for normal metabolism:** Metabolism helps control your weight and body temperature. Iron is needed to keep things humming properly.
- **Needed for proper development in infants and children:** Iron is particularly important during growth, and having enough ensures that the brain and body can fully develop.

- **Creation of hormones:** Iron makes myoglobin, a protein that is also used to make some hormones.
- **Optimal functioning of the immune system:** Keeping tissues full of oxygen allows for healthy functioning and proper cell turnover, which is key to a healthy immune system.
- **Conversion of beta-carotene to the active form of vitamin A:** Iron helps convert pro-vitamin A to the active form that your body can utilize.
- **Production of collagen:** Collagen holds body tissue together, and iron plus vitamin C help to synthesize it.

## Benefits

- **Boosts muscle function:** By ensuring that your muscles get enough oxygen, iron helps to keep them working as they should.
- **Improves mental acuity:** Iron is essential for bringing nourishing oxygen to your brain.
- **Improves energy:** Iron keeps you feeling energized and able to keep up with daily activities. One of the signs of low iron is always feeling tired.
- **Regulates body temperature:** Iron is needed for proper metabolism and body temperature. Always feeling cold can be a sign of iron deficiency.
- **Fights off infections as well as colds and flus:** Low iron makes your immune system weak and can cause you to get sick more frequently.
- **Improves focus:** Properly oxygenated brains have an easier time staying on task.

## Side Effects, Warnings, and Precautions

Many people know iron is really good for them, but not everyone realizes that too much iron is toxic. More and more research supports eating a more plant-based diet, and avoiding intake of too much iron (since the heme version from meat is more easily absorbed) is yet another reason why this is a good idea. It's also prudent to mention that even though your body naturally regulates iron absorption based on your needs, it's very difficult for your body to get rid of it.

A small number of people have a genetic condition called hemochromatosis, which causes high amounts of iron to be stored in the body. It can lead to organ damage and other problems. There are genetic tests available that can confirm the presence of this condition.

## Signs of Deficiency

Iron deficiency is both the most common mineral deficiency in the world and in the US, where an estimated 10 million people are iron deficient. Sometimes, it's necessary to take an iron supplement to boost low levels, but this should only be done for a set amount of time and not permanently. You should consult a registered dietitian if you need supplementation.

Because iron is lost in menstrual blood, teenage girls and women who menstruate tend to be at the highest risk for iron deficiency. As need for iron increases during pregnancy, this is another important time to ensure that intake is optimized. Children are also at risk of deficiency and iron anemia, especially if their mothers didn't consume enough and they were born with low stores.

Signs of deficiency can include:

- Feeling tired and weak
- Difficulty regulating body temperature and feeling cold
- Feeling light-headed/dizzy
- Headaches
- Inflammation of the tongue (glossitis)
- Frequent illness/infection

## How Much You Need (RDA)

| AGE | MALE | FEMALE |
| --- | --- | --- |
| 0–6 months (AI)* | 0.27mg | 0.27mg |
| 7–12 months | 11mg | 11mg |
| 1–3 years | 7mg | 7mg |
| 4–8 years | 10mg | 10mg |
| 9–13 years | 8mg | 8mg |
| 14–18 years | 11mg | 15mg |
| 19–50 years | 8mg | 18mg |
| 51+ years | 8mg | 8mg |
| Pregnancy | – | 27mg |
| Lactation | – | 9mg |

* Adequate Intake—this is the amount that babies receive from breast milk or formula, which is fortified with iron.

## Upper Limit (Amount Per Day)

| AGE | MALE | FEMALE |
|---|---|---|
| 0–6 months | 40mg | 40mg |
| 7–12 months | 40mg | 40mg |
| 1–3 years | 40mg | 40mg |
| 4–8 years | 40mg | 40mg |
| 9–13 years | 40mg | 40mg |
| 14–18 years | 45mg | 45mg |
| 19+ years | 45mg | 45mg |
| Pregnancy | – | 45mg |
| Lactation | – | 45mg |

## Best Way to Consume

Iron from the foods you eat isn't absorbed very efficiently; in other words, its bioavailability is low. While heme iron is more bioavailable than nonheme, only 15–35 percent of it actually gets absorbed. Nonheme is even lower, with only 5–12 percent getting absorbed. The RDA values do account for this, however, so as long as you're eating foods containing iron and boosting with vitamin C–rich foods to help the absorption, you can get enough.

Complicating things a little further are compounds in some foods that actually inhibit the absorption of iron. These include phytates (found in whole grains), some polyphenols, chlorogenic acid (found in coffee and cocoa), and tannins (found in tea). As long as you drink things like coffee, tea, and hot cocoa about an hour before or after eating, you can avoid many of these absorption-inhibiting effects. And on the flip side, remembering to include fruits and veggies (which contain vitamin C) *with* meals will help increase absorption.

Another interesting fact is that the darker the meat, the more iron it has! So if you want to get more iron naturally, choose dark-meat chicken or turkey over light. Beef liver will have much more iron than other cuts of beef. This is because iron (in the form of hemoglobin) gives the meat that deep red color.

## Natural Food Sources

### HEME FOOD SOURCES

| FOOD (SERVING SIZE) | IRON (MG) |
|---|---|
| Clams, cooked (3.2 ounces) | 28 (can vary depending on where clams are harvested) |
| Beef liver, pan fried (3 ounces) | 15 |
| Chicken liver, pan fried (3 ounces) | 13 |

| FOOD (SERVING SIZE) | IRON (MG) |
| --- | --- |
| Oysters, cooked with moist heat (3 ounces) | 8 |
| Sardines, canned in oil, drained (3 ounces) | 2 |
| Lean beef, cooked (3 ounces) | 2 |
| Chicken, roasted, meat and skin (3 ounces) | 1 |
| Tuna, canned in water, drained (3 ounces) | 1 |
| Turkey, roasted, meat and skin (3 ounces) | 1 |

## NONHEME FOOD SOURCES

| FOOD (SERVING SIZE) | IRON (MG) |
| --- | --- |
| White beans, canned, drained (1 cup) | 8 |
| Pumpkin seeds (2 tablespoons) | 4.2 |
| Pistachio nuts (1 cup) | 4.8 |
| Tofu, cubed (½ cup) | 3 |
| Spinach, boiled and drained (½ cup) | 3 |
| Quinoa, cooked (1 cup) | 2.8 |
| Chickpeas, boiled and drained (½ cup) | 2 |
| Cashew nuts, oil roasted (2 tablespoons) | 2 |
| Dark chocolate, 45–69% cacao solids (1 ounce) | 2 |
| Broccoli, chopped, boiled, drained (1 cup) | 1 |

# Asian-Inspired Beef and Broccoli with Peanuts *Serves 1*

This Asian dish is bursting with flavor. It is also an excellent source of iron and a great weeknight dinner option.

---

¼ tablespoon extra-virgin olive oil

¼ pound flank steak, cut into bite-sized pieces

½ medium shallot, peeled and chopped

1 medium green onion, chopped

1 clove garlic, chopped

2 tablespoons finely chopped peanuts

1 cup Chinese broccoli, chopped

½ tablespoon cornstarch

3 tablespoons water

2 teaspoons low-sodium soy sauce

½ tablespoon brown sugar

½ cup cooked brown rice

---

**PER SERVING**

*Calories: 493, Fat: 19g, Protein: 33g, Sodium: 352mg, Fiber: 5g, Carbohydrates: 44g, Sugar: 10g, Iron: 3.3mg*

1 Heat oil in a medium skillet over medium-high heat. Add beef and brown in the oil for about 5 minutes, then remove from heat. Set aside.

2 In the same pan, combine the shallot, green onion, garlic, and peanuts with the beef drippings. Stir frequently for 1 minute.

3 Add broccoli, then cover and cook 3–4 minutes.

4 In a small bowl, mix the cornstarch and water until they're smooth. Add soy sauce and sugar and stir until combined. Remove the lid from the skillet and add the sauce. Cook about 4 minutes or until sauce starts to thicken.

5 Add the beef back in and stir. Cook until warmed through.

6 Serve on top of brown rice.

# Vitamin K

Have you ever gotten a paper cut and noticed how quickly it stopped bleeding? That's thanks to vitamin K, which is responsible for blood clotting. This coagulation, or thickening of the blood when you begin to bleed, is what helps the bleeding to stop quickly. It's called vitamin K because upon its discovery by Danish researcher Henrik Dam, it was referred to as *Koagulationsvitamin* in a German journal. While this is the main and best-known role of vitamin K in the body, it actually has a number of other interesting and valuable functions that may surprise you.

## Description

Vitamin K is one of the few vitamins you can make. Well, you don't exactly make all of it—some of the good bacteria in your gut do. It's one of the reasons you should use caution with antibiotics—when you use them too frequently or over a long period of time, they can kill off some of the beneficial bugs in your gut and decrease the amount of vitamin K you have in your system.

Vitamin K can be found in two main forms: $K_1$ and $K_2$. Both are fat-soluble and naturally present in foods.

- $K_1$: plant-based foods such as greens, like spinach, Swiss chard, and kale
- $K_2$: fermented foods such as natto (a traditional Japanese food made from fermented soybeans) and some animal products like chicken, pork chops, and beef liver.

While there are plenty of foods that provide the two types of vitamin K, it has been estimated that up to half of the daily vitamin K requirement is provided by your gut bacteria.

## Role in the Body

- **Blood clotting:** Vitamin K helps to synthesize at least four of the thirteen factors in the blood that cause it to clot when you start to bleed, so that the bleeding stops quickly.
- **Controls calcium deposits:** Vitamin K helps calcium go where it's supposed to (bones) and not where it shouldn't (blood vessels).
- **Cell signaling and division:** Recent research has shown that vitamin K helps form components of cells that are responsible for helping to transmit signals in your nervous system and for proper cell division.

- **Assists in the formation of some nutrients that support the kidneys, bones, and blood:** Vitamin K works together with vitamin D to strengthen and support your bones. It is also involved in keeping your kidneys and blood healthy.

**Benefits**

- **Stops excessive bleeding and ensures wounds heal:** By ensuring that clotting factors can form quickly in response to an injury, vitamin K helps to stop bleeding and speed healing.
- **Reduces the risk of heart disease:** Hardening (i.e., calcification or deposits of calcium) of the arteries is one of the leading causes of heart disease. Vitamin K helps tell calcium where to go so it doesn't cause this dangerous condition.
- **May lower the risk of osteoporosis:** Some studies have shown that women who optimized their intake of vitamin K had lower risks of osteoporosis (weakened bones) and hip fractures.

**Side Effects, Warnings, and Precautions**

There is no upper limit set for vitamin K intake, but some people need to be cautious depending on medical conditions and medications, particularly blood thinners such as warfarin, which can have negative interactions with vitamin K.

**Signs of Deficiency**

Deficiency is rare in US adults, but it might occur in infants. This is due to their sterile GI tract, which means they have few bacteria for vitamin K production, and because of the lack of vitamin K in breast milk. People who use antibiotics might be at higher risk of vitamin K deficiency. Any individuals with disorders of fat and nutrient malabsorption such as cystic fibrosis, celiac disease, Crohn's disease, chronic pancreatitis, or liver disease, and people who have had intestinal bypass surgery, may be at risk of deficiency as well.

Signs of deficiency can include:

- Bruising easily
- Bleeding excessively (especially the gums or nose)
- Weakened bones

**How Much You Need**

No Recommended Daily Allowance has been set for vitamin K at this time and we don't know enough about $K_2$ to set a recommendation at all. Adequate Intake for $K_1$ is as follows:

| AGE | MALE | FEMALE |
|---|---|---|
| 0–6 months | 2mcg | 2mcg |
| 7–12 months | 2.5mcg | 2.5mcg |
| 1–3 years | 30mcg | 30mcg |
| 4–8 years | 55mcg | 55mcg |
| 9–13 years | 60mcg | 60mcg |
| 14–18 years | 75mcg | 75mcg |
| 19+ years | 120mcg | 90mcg |
| Pregnancy | – | 90mcg |
| Lactation | – | 90mcg |

## Best Way to Consume

It is ideal to consume fat-soluble vitamins like vitamin K with dietary fat to increase absorption. One way to achieve this is to consume dark leafy greens on most days and cook them in a little bit of olive oil to boost vitamin K intake. Many people don't get enough $K_2$, which is found in certain animal products and fermented foods. Try some of the fermented foods from the second list about once a week to get more $K_2$.

## Natural Food Sources

| FOOD (SERVING SIZE) | VITAMIN $K_1$ (MCG) |
|---|---|
| Collards, frozen, boiled (½ cup) | 530 |
| Turnipgreens, frozen, boiled (½ cup) | 426 |
| Mustardgreens, cooked (½ cup) | 415 |
| Spinach, raw (1 cup) | 145 |
| Kale, raw (1 cup) | 113 |
| Brussels sprouts (½ cup) | 109 |
| Okra, raw (½ cup) | 16 |
| Pine nuts, dried (1 ounce) | 15 |
| Grapes (½ cup) | 11 |

| FOOD (SERVING SIZE) | VITAMIN $K_2$ (MCG) |
|---|---|
| Natto (3 ounces) | 850 (the amount may vary depending on the strains of bacteria used) |
| Pork chop, cooked (3 ounces) | 59 |
| Chicken breast, meat only, cooked (3 ounces) | 13 |

| FOOD (SERVING SIZE) | VITAMIN K₂ (MCG) |
| --- | --- |
| Pumpkin, canned (½ cup) | 20 |
| Sauerkraut, raw (3 ounces) | 10 (the amount may vary depending on the strains of bacteria used) |
| Ground beef, broiled (3 ounces) | 6 |
| Chicken liver, braised (3 ounces) | 6 |
| Miso (1 tablespoon) | 5 (the amount may vary depending on the strains of bacteria used) |
| Egg, hard-boiled (1 large) | 4 |

## RECIPES

# Rice Bowl with Kimchi and Natto *Serves 1*

The natto in this recipe is high in vitamin K₂. Natto is a popular food in Japan and it's made out of fermented soybeans. Kimchi is fermented cabbage. Together these foods make for a great flavor combination and vitamin boost.

1 small head bok choy, chopped

½ cup steamed brown rice

½ cup kimchi

1 large egg

1 tablespoon natto

Handful mung bean sprouts

1 tablespoon low-sodium soy sauce

1 sheet nori

1 teaspoon hot sauce

**PER SERVING**
*Calories: 376, Fat: 10g, Protein: 28g, Sodium: 1,466mg, Fiber: 13g, Carbohydrates: 52g, Sugar: 13g*

1 Arrange bok choy, rice, and kimchi in a bowl.
2 In a small skillet, fry the egg to your liking and add on top of rice bowl.
3 Top with natto, sprouts, and soy sauce. Break the nori sheet apart and sprinkle on top.
4 Add hot sauce, and serve.

# Tuscan Kale Soup  *Serves 3*

This recipe is high in vitamin K₁ and is a great dinner option for busier weeks. Make a large pot and freeze some for a quick and healthy meal. Serve this soup with some whole-wheat bread to boost the fiber.

¼ medium yellow onion, peeled and diced

½ tablespoon extra-virgin olive oil

1 clove garlic, minced

¼ teaspoon turmeric

3 cups low-sodium vegetable broth

¼ cup lentils

1 medium stalk celery, chopped

1 small sweet potato, peeled and chopped

1 small carrot, peeled and chopped

1 small zucchini, chopped

1 cup canned diced tomatoes

1 teaspoon dried oregano

½ teaspoon crushed red pepper

Pinch salt

Pinch black pepper

1 cup chopped kale

1 sprig fresh thyme

**PER SERVING**

*Calories: 174, Fat: 3g, Protein: 8g, Sodium: 432mg, Fiber: 7g, Carbohydrates: 32g, Sugar: 11g, Vitamin K: 1.5g*

1  In a large stockpot, sauté onions in oil 3–5 minutes. Add garlic and turmeric and cook another 1–2 minutes.
2  Add broth and bring to a boil.
3  Add the remaining ingredients, except for the kale and thyme. Let simmer 40 minutes.
4  Add kale and fresh thyme and cook 5 minutes, or until kale is wilted.
5  Serve immediately.

# Magnesium

The wide-ranging, positive effects of magnesium cannot be overstated. Yet, recent estimates indicate that 50–80 percent of the US population isn't getting enough of this phenomenal nutrient. Depletion of our soil, weakening of our gut health through chronic overuse of medications like painkillers and antibiotics, as well as diets high in processed foods are the main culprits in our nationwide magnesium deficiency. It's time to course-correct and start including more magnesium in our diets. Fortunately, it's actually pretty easy to eat magnesium-rich foods throughout the day to meet your needs, when you know which foods to include.

## Description

There are seven essential minerals that humans require in high doses. Magnesium is one of these "macro minerals." Most of it is stored in your bones, tissues, and muscle, and a small amount floats around in the blood and other fluids. Did you know that every single cell in your body has magnesium in it? Magnesium guides the reactivity process of more than three hundred different key functions that are constantly occurring to keep you healthy and alive.

These functions include everything from making energy, synthesizing protein, and supporting gene transcription to maintaining muscle function, including the heart muscle, plus much more.

As more research comes out on magnesium, we're learning that it is also linked to conditions such as diabetes, heart disease, depression and anxiety, sleep disorders, chronic pain, and blood pressure. Some researchers even believe that the climbing rates of mood disorders in our society might be partly linked to the fact that we're not eating enough magnesium-rich foods.

## Role in the Body

- **Bone health:** Magnesium helps pull calcium into bones and works to increase bone density, thus preventing osteoporosis. Magnesium also helps to activate vitamin D inside the kidneys, so it can do its own work inside the body.
- **Enzymatic functioning:** Hundreds and hundreds of different enzymes rely on magnesium to guide them to take correct action in multitudes of areas throughout the body.
- **Carbohydrate and sugar processing:** Sufficient amounts of magnesium

are needed to properly manage the breakdown and metabolism of carbs and sugars, as well as proper insulin function.

- **Muscle movement:** Magnesium is essential for the relaxation and contraction of your muscles. Athletes and people who are highly active need extra magnesium.
- **Blood pressure:** Magnesium helps to control blood pressure, and a balanced diet including enough magnesium can manage blood pressure and help blood vessels to relax properly.
- **Neurotransmitter balance:** Magnesium affects brain function and mood. Magnesium deficiency has been linked with increased risk of depression.

## Benefits

- **Promotes heart health:** Studies have shown an association between higher blood levels of magnesium and lower risk of heart disease.
- **Alleviates depression:** Research indicates that people with depression, anxiety, and other mental health disorders tend to have much lower levels of magnesium. Some studies have shown that boosting magnesium levels may be as effective as antidepressant medication in some people.
- **Enhances athletic performance:** Athletes require sufficient levels of

magnesium to optimize their performance (and often need increased magnesium depending on their activity level).

- **Alleviates migraine headaches:** Keeping magnesium at healthy levels may help to prevent headaches and migraines.
- **Lessens PMS symptoms:** Magnesium may help to reduce symptoms of premenstrual disorder in women, including bloating, headaches, dizziness, and sugar cravings.
- **Regulates sleep cycle:** There are well-established links between magnesium and sleep cycles. Increasing magnesium intake may help regulate sleep, which is critical for so many other aspects of physical and mental health.
- **Aids with digestion:** Sufficient magnesium is important for healthy bowel movements and can help to relieve or prevent constipation.

## Side Effects, Warnings, and Precautions

Getting too much magnesium from foods isn't a concern because the body will naturally excrete any extra to keep the right balance. However, it is possible to get too much magnesium from supplements, which can cause side effects such as diarrhea, nausea, vomiting, and weakness. A severe overdose can result in respiratory distress and abnormal heartbeat.

Also, magnesium supplements have been shown to interact with many medications, including antibiotics, diuretics, and heart health drugs, so it's very important to check with your doctor and dietitian before starting supplements.

## Signs of Deficiency

Signs of deficiency can include:

- **Trouble sleeping:** Magnesium plays an important role in maintaining GABA, a neurotransmitter that promotes deep sleep.
- **Anxiety/mood disorders:** Since magnesium contributes to brain function and signaling, magnesium deficiency may increase risk of anxiety, mood disorders, and depression.
- **Fatigue, weakness:** Fatigue— physical and mental exhaustion— and muscle weakness may be linked to magnesium deficiency.
- **Numbness, cramping, tingling, and seizures:** Severe magnesium deficiency (which is very rare) may lead to numbness, twitching, tremors, and muscle cramps.
- **Abnormal heartbeat:** Very low levels of magnesium can cause abnormal heartbeat since magnesium helps maintain a healthy heart rhythm.

## How Much You Need (RDA)

| AGE | MALE | FEMALE |
| --- | --- | --- |
| 0–6 months | 30mg (AI) | 30mg (AI) |
| 7–12 months | 75mg (AI) | 75mg (AI) |
| 1–3 years | 80mg | 80mg |
| 4–8 years | 130mg | 130mg |
| 9–13 years | 240mg | 240mg |
| 14–18 years | 410mg | 360mg |
| 19–30 years | 400mg | 310mg |
| 31–50 years | 420mg | 320mg |
| 51+ years | 420mg | 320mg |
| Pregnancy | – | 350–360mg |
| Lactation | – | 310–320mg |

## Tolerable Upper Intake Levels for Supplemental Magnesium (Amount Per Day)

| AGE | MALE | FEMALE |
| --- | --- | --- |
| 0–12 months | Not established | Not established |
| 1–3 years | 65mg | 65mg |
| 4–8 years | 110mg | 110mg |
| 9–18 years | 350mg | 350mg |
| 19+ years | 350mg | 350mg |
| Pregnancy | – | 350mg |
| Lactation | – | 350mg |

## Best Way to Consume

Magnesium has limited bioavailability, so it's important to consume adequate amounts on most days or, ideally, every day. A great way to do this is to snack on a handful of nuts and seeds (especially sunflower seeds), which are great sources of magnesium plus lots of other healthy nutrients. Magnesium is the central ion inside of chlorophyll, the compound that gives plants their green color, so green leafy vegetables tend to contain a good amount of magnesium and are also highly nutrient-dense.

## Natural Food Sources

| FOOD (SERVING SIZE) | MAGNESIUM (MG) |
| --- | --- |
| Sunflower seeds (½ cup) | 228 |
| Pumpkin seeds (½ cup) | 176 |
| Almonds, dry roasted (1 ounce) | 80 |
| Spinach, cooked (½ cup) | 78 |
| Cashews, dry roasted (1 ounce) | 74 |
| Peanuts, oil roasted (¼ cup) | 63 |
| Black beans, cooked (½ cup) | 60 |
| Edamame, shelled, cooked (½ cup) | 50 |
| Avocado, peeled, pitted, cubed (1 cup) | 44 |
| Potato, baked with skin (3½ ounces) | 43 |

# Green Machine Morning Smoothie *Serves 1*

This smoothie is a great source of magnesium and other nutrients! It's a perfect to-go breakfast for those who don't have a lot of time in the morning.

---

1 medium frozen banana, peeled

1 cup macadamia milk

¼ cup frozen mango chunks

1 cup fresh spinach

¼ medium avocado, peeled, pitted, and sliced

2 tablespoons sunflower seeds

Ice, as needed

---

**PER SERVING**

*Calories: 328, Fat: 18g, Protein: 7g, Sodium: 121mg, Fiber: 10g, Carbohydrates: 42g, Sugar: 20g, Magnesium: 104mg*

Add all ingredients to a blender and mix until smooth. Add 1–2 ice cubes as desired.

# Manganese

Manganese is part of the essential trace mineral group. The name "manganese" is derived from the Greek word for "magic," which is very fitting, as this mineral has numerous important functions and catalyzes so many critical reactions that it could be considered almost miraculous. There's also some mystery surrounding manganese, as more research is needed to fully understand the diverse roles it plays in the body and what happens if you get too little or too much. Read on to understand why it's so beneficial to optimize your manganese intake and what foods to get it from.

## Description

Manganese activates numerous enzymes (compounds that speed up reactions inside your body) that are needed for metabolism, antioxidant functioning, bone development, collagen formation, and more. It also seems to be implicated in the prevention of chronic disease. While more research is needed to understand the mechanisms behind this, deficiency or suboptimal levels of manganese seem to be linked to conditions like diabetes and osteoporosis.

Some manganese is stored in your kidneys, liver, pancreas, and bones, but this isn't enough to meet your body's needs. You still need to get manganese from food sources. Some of the best sources of manganese are whole-grain products and certain vegetables and fruits, like sweet potato and pineapple.

## Role in the Body

- **Part of a powerful antioxidant:** Manganese is a component of the highly powerful antioxidant enzyme called manganese superoxide dismutase (MnSOD), which works inside of your mitochondria (where energy is produced!) to reduce cell damage caused by the by-products of energy production and oxygen.
- **Metabolism of carbs, proteins, and fats:** By combining with other compounds that help to break down foods into tiny molecules that can be used by the body, manganese helps to digest, or metabolize, your macronutrients (proteins, carbohydrates, and fats).
- **Assists with the formation of bones:** In combination with some other minerals, manganese supports bone formation and bone density.
- **Helps with collagen formation:** Collagen synthesis requires the amino acid proline, and to make proline, you need manganese.

- **Serves as a helper in numerous chemical processes in the body:** By combining with various enzymes, manganese helps to ensure that key processes in the body occur efficiently.
- **Necessary for proper brain function:** Helps protect the brain from free radical (damaging) molecules and also helps to activate some neurotransmitters that help electrical signals to pass more quickly in the body.

## Benefits

- **Can help to lower inflammation:** As part of the powerful antioxidant MnSOD, manganese helps to reduce cell damage from harmful compounds called free radicals, thus lowering inflammation.
- **May help to regulate blood sugar levels:** Some studies have shown that people with diabetes seem to have lower blood levels of manganese, but it's not yet fully clear if the low levels lead to issues with blood sugar, or if it's the other way around.
- **Possibly helps to reduce PMS symptoms in women:** One study indicated that when combined with calcium, manganese helped to decrease PMS symptoms in women.
- **Keeps your thyroid healthy:** Manganese helps to make thyroxine, a hormone that is key for normal thyroid functioning.
- **Assists in wound healing:** Wounds require extra collagen to heal quickly. Manganese is needed for collagen production, so that there's enough of it for healing, when necessary.

## Side Effects, Warnings, and Precautions

Too much manganese is toxic, but it's nearly impossible to get too much of this mineral from foods. Inhaled manganese dust is a neurotoxin (a poison that affects the nervous system) and can be inhaled by people working with metals, such as welders, and by those working in manganese mines. The early symptoms of manganese toxicity are irritability, aggressiveness, and hallucinations. Symptoms progress to tremors and spasms.

## Signs of Deficiency

Manganese deficiency is rare, but people who don't eat sufficient amounts of whole grains, vegetables, and fruits can experience suboptimal levels.

Signs of deficiency may include:

- Lowered cholesterol levels
- Temporary skin rash
- Elevated blood levels of calcium and phosphorous
- Elevated blood sugar levels

## How Much You Need

There is not enough data currently to set a Recommended Daily Allowance (RDA) for manganese. However, both an Adequate Intake (AI) recommendation and an Upper Intake Level (UL), which is the highest level per day that is estimated to pose zero risk, have been set.

## Adequate Intake (AI)

| AGE | MALE | FEMALE |
| --- | --- | --- |
| 0–6 months | 0.003mg | 0.003mg |
| 7–12 months | 0.6mg | 0.6mg |
| 1–3 years | 1.2mg | 1.2mg |
| 4–8 years | 1.5mg | 1.5mg |
| 9–13 years | 1.9mg | 1.6mg |
| 14–18 years | 2.2mg | 1.6mg |
| 19+ years | 2.3mg | 1.8mg |
| Pregnancy | – | 2.0mg |
| Lactation | – | 2.6mg |

## Upper Intake Level (UL)

| AGE | MALE | FEMALE |
| --- | --- | --- |
| 0–6 months | ND (not determined) | ND (not determined) |
| 7–12 months | ND (not determined) | ND (not determined) |
| 1–3 years | 2mg | 2mg |
| 4–8 years | 3mg | 3mg |
| 9–13 years | 6mg | 6mg |
| 14–18 years | 9mg | 9mg |
| 19+ years | 11mg | 11mg |
| Pregnancy | – | 11mg |
| Lactation | – | 11mg |

## Best Way to Consume

Manganese is found in plant-based foods, but the amount will vary depending on the health of the soil and how much manganese was absorbed by the plant. Some foods that contain manganese also contain compounds that slow down its absorption somewhat. These foods are nuts, seeds, beans, and whole grains, which contain phytic acid, and also foods that contain oxalic acid, which include spinach, kale, and Swiss chard.

## Natural Food Sources

| FOOD (SERVING SIZE) | MANGANESE (MG) |
| --- | --- |
| Oats, raw (¼ cup) | 1.92 |
| Pumpkin seeds (¼ cup) | 1.47 |
| Tofu, soft, cubed (4 ounces) | 1.34 |
| Pecans (19 halves) | 1.28 |
| Brown rice, cooked (½ cup) | 1.07 |
| Wheat germ, crude (1 tablespoon) | 0.95 |
| Spinach, cooked (½ cup) | 0.84 |
| Pineapple chunks, raw (½ cup) | 0.77 |
| Almonds (23 whole) | 0.65 |
| Sweet potato, cooked, mashed (½ cup) | 0.50 |

## RECIPE

# Green Bulgur Bowl  *Serves 1*

This bowl is fully plant-based and satisfying. Wheat germ and tofu are great sources of manganese and protein.

1 tablespoon extra-virgin olive oil

1 clove garlic, minced

¼ cup chopped onion

3 ounces tofu, cubed

½ cup chopped carrots

1 cup chopped savoy cabbage

½ cup cooked bulgur wheat

2 tablespoons chopped fresh parsley

1 tablespoon chopped almonds

Pinch salt

**PER SERVING**

*Calories: 370, Fat: 21g, Protein: 15g, Sodium: 372mg, Fiber: 11g, Carbohydrates: 36g, Sugar: 7g, Manganese: 1.6mg*

1  Heat oil in a medium skillet over medium heat and add garlic, onion, tofu, and carrots. Cook 3–4 minutes.

2  Add cabbage and cook another 3–4 minutes or until wilted.

3  Serve over bulgur wheat and garnish with parsley and almonds. Add salt. Enjoy!

# MCT and LCT

Medium-chain triglycerides (MCTs) and long-chain triglycerides (LCTs) are types of saturated fat. Saturated and unsaturated refers to the type of chemical structure the fat has. This chemical structure affects the way it acts and functions in your body. Some fats have mostly beneficial effects, while others have neutral or harmful effects. In general, saturated fats are definitely the less healthy type of fat—you can easily identify them because they are solid at room temperature, though not all saturated fats function in the same way, as you'll see further on in this chapter. Some examples of saturated fats include butter, lard, and coconut oil. Most saturated fats come from animal products. While it is commonly thought that saturated fat increases the risk of heart attack and stroke, more recent studies have begun to call this into question.

## Description

Fats are the most calorie-rich foods you eat, providing a lot of energy and many other benefits as well as some potential downsides. Aside from being such a dense energy source, the many different types of fats have varying roles in the body. They help make up cells and tissues; for example, your brain is made up of about 60 percent fat, and fat is a component of every cell in the body. Fats are also used in the production of hormones and to help transport all of the fat-soluble vitamins (A, D, E, and K). That's why people who are on a very low-fat diet may have low vitamin levels as well. Fats also have qualities that make food taste delicious and that help your taste buds and brains to feel satisfied after meals.

## Role in the Body

- **Absorbing and bringing vitamins to the tissues where they are needed:** All of the fat-soluble vitamins (A, D, E, and K) rely on fats to help them get absorbed and transported to where they need to go.
- **Formation of hormones:** Fat cells are an important part of the body's endocrine system, which makes hormones. These hormones help to regulate blood sugar, blood pressure, muscle contractions, and more.
- **Immune system functioning:** Fats are critical to your immune system. They can either upregulate it to be more efficient and effective, as is the case with many of the unsaturated fats, or they can downregulate and

cause it to be weaker, which is what happens when you get too many saturated fats in your diet. Over time, researchers have found that these effects can induce or reduce chronic conditions like diabetes, heart disease, and others.

## Benefits

- Adequate formation and functioning of hormones
- Optimization of fat-soluble vitamin levels
- Improved ability to fight off infections and illness
- Satisfaction and pleasurable meal experience
- Reduced inflammation (specifically MCTs)
- Brain and eye health and good functioning, and protection from degeneration

## Side Effects, Warnings, and Precautions

Too much fat can be just as harmful as too little. It's an essential nutrient that can keep you healthy and reduce the risk of disease when in the right balance. Consuming too much fat, especially saturated fat, can lead to negative health consequences. Inflammation, increased lipid levels, heart disease, and weight gain are some of the negative side effects of excess fats. Saturated and trans fats in particular have been linked to heart disease and a rise in "bad" cholesterol levels.

## Signs of Deficiency

Avoiding fat is a bad idea. Some people go on very low-fat diets in an attempt to lose weight, but this can often backfire and lead to overeating, as fat is necessary for the satiety mechanisms and enjoyment of food. Too little fat tissue in the body can also cause problems and affect hormone production, immunity, and heart health. People with certain medical conditions like HIV/AIDS, cystic fibrosis, and anorexia nervosa are at a higher risk of becoming deficient in fat. People who have digestive conditions and absorption problems may also have a hard time eating enough fats or absorbing them. In these specific cases, supplementation with an easily absorbable fat like MCT oil may be warranted and helpful.

Signs of deficiency can include:

- Low vitamin levels
- Inflammation
- Increased risk of heart disease
- Improper cell function/increased cell damage
- Disruption of endocrine system/hormone production

- Difficulty getting pregnant/fertility issues/loss of menstruation
- Dry and weak skin, hair, and nails

## How Much You Need

Genetics play a role in fat intake. Not everyone responds to fats in exactly the same way. Some people actually need a bit more fat, while others need a bit less. This means that your intake of fats may be slightly different from someone else's, though there are good general guidelines that apply to almost everyone.

The following table lists the healthy ranges of total fats and saturated fats that you should aim for daily, depending on your calorie intake. If you're not sure what your calorie intake should be, meet with a registered dietitian to get your personal amounts calculated.

| BASED ON CALORIE CONSUMPTION | YOUR ADMR* FOR DAILY TOTAL FAT IS 20–35% OF CALORIES | YOU SHOULD LIMIT YOUR DAILY SATURATED FAT TO 5–6% OF CALORIES** |
|---|---|---|
| 1,000 | 22–39g | 5.5–6.6g |
| 1,200 | 26.6–46.6g | 6.6–8g |
| 1,400 | 31–54g | 7.8–9.3g |
| 1,600 | 36–62g | 8.8–10.6g |
| 2,000 | 44–78g | 11–13.3g |
| 2,200 | 49–86g | 12.2–14.6g |
| 2,500 | 56–97g | 13.8–16.6g |
| 2,800 | 62–109g | 15.5–18.6g |

* Acceptable Macronutrient Distribution Range. These numbers reflect the 2015–2020 Dietary Guidelines for Americans.

* *The American Heart Association recommends limiting saturated fats to 5–6 percent of daily intake. The 2015–2020 Dietary Guidelines for Americans recommend less than 10 percent.

## Best Way to Consume

Contrary to past dietary advice, a low-fat diet is not necessarily healthy. Research has shown that the issue is much more complex and nuanced. The quality of fats and the other macronutrients (such as carbohydrates and protein) matter just as much as quantity.

While it's important to limit saturated fats, it's equally important that you replace them with good fats—the unsaturated ones—and not refined carbohydrates, which include such foods as white bread, processed crackers, chips, and cookies. Research has also shown that not all saturated fats function exactly the same way. For example, coconut oil is a saturated fat, but it has more medium-chain triglycerides (MCTs) than the saturated fat that comes from animal products. MCTs are healthier than other saturated fats and may even help with weight loss, satiety, inflammation, and more. However, the bottom line is that all saturated fats should be minimized.

Getting plant-based sources of fats (with the exception of fish for omega-3s) is a good way to get the best types of fats in your diet while minimizing the harmful ones. Focus on foods like olive oil, nuts, seeds, and avocados. Reduce things that are high in saturated fats like fast food, meat (especially red meat), pizza, cheese, butter, and high-fat dairy desserts.

## Natural Food Sources

| FOOD (SERVING SIZE) | SATURATED FAT (G) |
| --- | --- |
| Beef fat (tallow) (3½ ounces) | 50 |
| Lamb, rib roast, roasted (3½ ounces) | 15 |
| Coconut oil (1 tablespoon) | 12 |
| 70%ground beef, 30% fat (3½ ounces) | 11 |
| Pork, spareribs, braised (3½ ounces) | 8 |
| Poultry with skin (3½ ounces) | 7 |
| Butter (1 tablespoon) | 7 |
| Lard (1 tablespoon) | 5 |

| FOOD (SERVING SIZE) | TOTAL FAT | MCT CONTENT |
| --- | --- | --- |
| Coconut oil (1 tablespoon) | 14g | Greater than 60% |
| Palm kernel oil (1 tablespoon) | 14g | Greater than 50% |
| Butter (1 tablespoon) | 12g | 6.8% |
| Cheddar cheese (1 ounce) | 9g | 7.3% |
| Full-fat yogurt (8 ounces) | 7.4g | 6.6% |

## RECIPE

# Peachy Keen Coconut Smoothie *Serves 1*

Here's a recipe that contains both heart-healthy monounsaturated fats and some MCTs, balanced out with the other macronutrients (protein and carbs) for a delicious and heart-healthy snack.

| | | |
| --- | --- | --- |
| ¼ medium avocado, peeled, pitted, and sliced | ½ cup frozen peach slices | 1 tablespoon pumpkin seeds |
| ½ cup blueberries | ½ cup light coconut milk | Ice, as needed |

**PER SERVING**
*Calories: 220, Fat: 12g, Protein: 3g, Sodium: 9mg, Fiber: 6g, Carbohydrates: 25g, Sugar: 14g*

Add all ingredients to a blender and mix until smooth, adding ice as desired. Enjoy!

# Molybdenum

Never heard of molybdenum? Many people have no idea what this essential mineral does or what foods to get it from. It's one of the trace minerals, meaning you need it in very small amounts. Even though you don't need much of it, it plays a large role in your body's detox pathways, helping to get rid of toxins and wastes. Researchers have even hypothesized that it may have played a key role in evolution, as it's essential for a key step in nitrogen conversion, which is what helped single-celled organisms evolve millions of years ago into the wide array of animals and plants that exist today.

## Description

Soil throughout the earth contains varying levels of molybdenum, and it gets into your system when you consume plants grown in molybdenum-rich soil as well as certain animal products. Molybdenum works as a cofactor in the body and turns on at least four different essential enzymes (you can think of them as helper molecules) to break down toxins and toxic waste products of metabolism, and to activate antioxidants.

One of the key functions of molybdenum is sulfate breakdown, which helps to prevent the dangerous buildup of sulfites that come from foods and added preservatives. Sulfite buildup can lead to allergic reactions in some people such as skin rash, diarrhea, and breathing problems.

## Role in the Body

- **Detoxification:** Molybdenum acts as a cofactor for four different important enzymes that help to package up and move waste products and toxins out of the body.
- **Prevents buildup of sulfites in the body:** Molybdenum helps to convert sulfite to sulfate, which is a mineral salt and can be excreted so that sulfites don't build up in the blood.
- **Helps with the metabolism of amino acids:** Molybdenum specifically works with the two sulfur-containing amino acids, methionine and cysteine, which are the building blocks of some proteins.
- **Partners with riboflavin:** Molybdenum works with vitamin $B_2$ to incorporate iron into hemoglobin.

## Benefits

- Helps your body to flush out toxins and waste products

- Helps the liver to break down alcohol and some medicines, such as cancer therapy drugs
- Prevents anemia by optimizing iron storage and by assisting riboflavin in using iron to create red blood cells

## Side Effects, Warnings, and Precautions

There are no positive health effects of taking too much molybdenum; in fact, in large amounts, such as those that you could get from supplements, it can be harmful. Very high intakes of molybdenum (10,000–15,000 micrograms) have been linked to conditions such as excess buildup of uric acid that causes gout-like symptoms. Also, high intake of molybdenum has been associated with poor bone growth and decreased fertility. When there's too much molybdenum in the body, it seems to compete with copper and blocks its absorption. In some rare cases, high consumption has caused seizures and brain damage. Excess molybdenum is typically excreted through urine.

## Signs of Deficiency

Your body stores some molybdenum in the liver and kidneys, and you get plenty from your food supply, so deficiency is very rare in healthy people. With a normal diet, there is no need to worry about molybdenum deficiency.

It has been observed that long-term deficiency may be linked to increased cases of esophageal cancer. In extremely rare cases, infants develop molybdenum cofactor deficiency, which is an unusual genetic condition that prevents them from activating the four enzymes that rely on molybdenum; this can lead to serious brain damage and seizures.

Signs of deficiency can include:

- Headaches
- Seizures
- Brain issues/disorders
- Visual disorders

## How Much You Need (AI)

| AGE | MALE | FEMALE |
| --- | --- | --- |
| 0–6 months | 2mcg | 2mcg |
| 7–12 months | 3mcg | 3mcg |
| 1–3 years | 17mcg | 17mcg |
| 4–8 years | 22mcg | 22mcg |
| 9–13 years | 34mcg | 34mcg |
| 14–18 years | 43mcg | 43mcg |
| 19+ years | 45mcg | 45mcg |
| Pregnancy | – | 50mcg |
| Lactation | – | 50mcg |

## Upper Limits (Amount Per Day)

| AGE | MALE | FEMALE |
| --- | --- | --- |
| 0–6 months | – | – |
| 7–12 months | – | – |
| 1–3 years | 0.3mg | 0.3mg |
| 4–8 years | 0.6mg | 0.6mg |
| 9–13 years | 1.1mg | 1.1mg |
| 14–18 years | 1.7mg | 1.7mg |
| 19+ years | 2mg | 2mg |
| Pregnancy | – | 2mg |
| Lactation | – | 2mg |

## Best Way to Consume

Eating just half a cup of beans or oats is more than enough to meet your daily requirements for molybdenum. Most whole grains and nuts also contain a good amount. The actual amount of molybdenum in foods, including those in the following table, is hard to estimate and will vary depending on the content of molybdenum in the soil the food is grown in.

## Natural Food Sources

| FOOD (SERVING SIZE) | MOLYBDENUM (MCG) |
| --- | --- |
| Mung beans (½ cup) | 410 |
| Lentils, dried, raw (1 cup) | 180 |
| Dried peas (1 cup) | 147 |
| Kidney beans (1 cup) | 133 |
| Lima beans, boiled (1 cup) | 104 |
| Oats, raw (¼ cup) | 29 |
| Peanuts (¼ cup) | 11 |
| Tomatoes, chopped (1 cup) | 9 |
| Walnuts (¼ cup) | 9 |
| Green peas, fresh (1 cup) | 7 |

# Nourishing Mung Bean Salad *Serves 2*

This salad is super satisfying and a great way to naturally boost your detoxifying mechanisms with both molybdenum and fiber.

| | | |
|---|---|---|
| 1 cup mung beans, cooked | ¼ medium red onion, peeled and sliced | 1 tablespoon chopped fresh cilantro |
| ½ cup peas | ¼ cup chopped walnuts | ½ teaspoon red pepper flakes |
| ½ cup cooked quinoa | 1 tablespoon extra-virgin olive oil | |
| 1 small tomato, cubed | Juice of ½ medium lime | ⅛ teaspoon black pepper |

**PER SERVING**
*Calories: 322, Fat: 14g, Protein: 14g, Sodium: 8mg, Fiber: 12g, Carbohydrates: 38g, Sugar: 6g*

1 In a large bowl, combine mung beans, peas, quinoa, tomato, onion, and walnuts.
2 In a small bowl, mix oil with lime juice, cilantro, red pepper, and black pepper, and then drizzle over salad. Serve.

# Omega-3

Omega-3s have been said to cure cancer, prevent heart disease, alleviate depression and anxiety, extend your life span, and much more. But what's true and what's not? Not all of these claims are substantiated by research, and some of the studies on omega-3 have come back with mixed results, while others show some promising benefits. There are also interesting observations on the differences in benefits when getting whole-food sources of omegas versus taking supplements. The truth is, there's a lot we still don't know about these fatty acids. Let's review what we do know and sift through the hype and reality and look at some of the best ways to get these essential nutrients into your diet.

## Description

There are three main types of omega-3 fatty acids: alpha-linolenic acid (ALA), docosahexaenoic acid (DHA), and eicosapentaenoic acid (EPA). There is also a fourth omega-3 called eicosatetraenoic acid (ETA), which is only found in a few, unique foods like roe oil. Your body needs omega-3s to function properly and prevent disease.

Omega-3s are part of the unsaturated fats family. Specifically, these are all polyunsaturated fatty acids. "Poly" means "many," and "unsaturated" refers to the type of chemical bond they form. So, these fatty acids have "many unsaturated bonds." The difference between them is the length of their chemical chains. Alpha-linolenic acid (ALA) has a shorter chain, while DHA and EPA have longer chains. The length of these chains affects what they do inside your body. ALA is found in certain plant foods, like walnuts, chia seeds, and flaxseeds. DHA and EPA are found mostly in oily fish, such as herring, trout, and mackerel. It's important to consume a mix of foods that contain these fatty acids because your body can't make them on its own.

Some of omega-3's most important functions are related to heart health, hormone production, and brain development. Research is being conducted on these fatty acids to better understand exactly how much we need and the various roles they play. Long-term studies consistently show that people with higher fish and seafood intakes have better health than those who consume less fish and more meat. While more research is needed to determine why this is, it's thought that omega-3s are a contributing factor, though the other nutrients in seafood like vitamins, minerals, and other compounds also likely play a role.

## Role in the Body

- **Reduction of inflammation:** EPA helps form messenger molecules called eicosanoids, which help to reduce inflammation.
- **Depression:** EPA also helps with mental health, particularly depression. One study showed that it may be as effective as an antidepressant.
- **Lowering unhealthy fat levels in the blood:** Omega-3s can help lower a type of fat called triglycerides and are even prescribed by doctors for this use. However, data on whether they improve heart health is mixed; numerous studies have shown that the supplemental form does not have a substantial effect, while others have shown slight benefits in certain populations, but especially when the omegas come from food sources like fish.
- **Protection and strengthening of skin:** The structural parts of your skin cells require DHA to stay plump and soft, and require EPA to stay hydrated, smooth, and acne-free. Both DHA and EPA help to prevent wrinkles and reduce sun damage.
- **Supporting your body to fall and stay asleep:** Omega-3s help produce compounds that are needed for good-quality rest.
- **May play a role in cancer protection:** Some studies have shown a link between increased intake of omega-3s and cancer, but not all studies are in agreement. It seems that diets higher in fatty fish may reduce the risk of some cancers.
- **Building blocks for brain, nerve, and eye cells:** Almost half of the fats in your brain are made up of DHA. It's especially important for nerve and eye cells and can help prevent an eye problem called macular degeneration.
- **Essential for proper brain development in babies:** Studies have shown that increased DHA is linked to increased IQ scores and a decreased risk of some diseases.
- **Brain health:** Some studies have linked eating more fish to a lower risk of dementia and Alzheimer's disease.

While more studies are needed, it seems that omega-3s may also play a role in prevention or reduction of allergies, attention deficit hyperactivity disorder, and numerous other health conditions.

## Benefits

- Improved lipid (fat) levels in the blood; may help reduce the risk of heart disease
- Reduction of depression, anxiety, and possibly other mental health disorders
- Reduction of inflammation
- Clear, healthy, well-hydrated skin

- Help with good quality sleep
- May reduce the risk of some cancers
- May help to reduce some of the pain and swelling associated with arthritis
- Help maintaining eye and brain health
- Promoting healthy development of babies
- May reduce menstrual pain

## Side Effects, Warnings, and Precautions

Most of us don't eat enough omega-3s. As with many other nutrients, you should focus on whole-food sources, especially sustainably raised fish. If you don't like fish, you can take a supplement to make sure you're getting enough of these valuable fatty acids. Just be aware that the supplement form may not be as effective as the food form. It's also possible to overdo it, so don't take more than the recommended amount on the label. Taking too many omega-3s in supplement form can cause the following side effects:

- Bad breath, strange taste in the mouth
- Upset stomach
- Nausea and vomiting
- Diarrhea
- Stinky sweat
- Headaches
- Heartburn

## Signs of Deficiency

People who don't consume fish twice a week or take supplemental omega-3s are at risk for deficiency or imbalance in their omega-3 to omega-6 ratio. Many Americans eat too many omega-6s and too few omega-3s, and this unbalanced ratio has been linked to increased inflammation and other health issues.

Also, people who have problems with absorption, especially fat absorption, may not be getting enough omega-3s and other fats.

Signs of deficiency can include:

- Dry, flaky, or peeling skin
- Skin patches and dullness
- Dandruff or dry, itchy scalp
- Dry mouth, throat, or eyes
- Joint pain, swelling, and inflammation

## How Much You Need

Alpha-linolenic acid (ALA) is the only omega-3 for which official RDA values have been established in the US. We know that DHA and EPA are essential as well, but there is no RDA amount for them yet, as more research is needed. However, global organizations like the World Health Organization (WHO) have recommended levels of 250–500 milligrams of both EPA and DHA for adults daily. While the American Heart Association doesn't give specific amounts, it does recommend eating about 3½ ounces of fatty fish at least twice a week to get enough omega-3s. Pregnant and breastfeeding women should get an extra 200 milligrams of DHA daily.

| AGE | MALE | FEMALE |
|---|---|---|
| 0–12 months* | 0.5g | 0.5g |
| 1–3 years | 0.7g | 0.7g |
| 4–8 years | 0.9g | 0.9g |
| 9–13 years | 1.2g | 1.0g |
| 14–18 years | 1.6g | 1.1g |
| 19+ years | 1.6g | 1.1g |
| Pregnancy | – | 1.4g |
| Lactation | – | 1.3g |

\* Total omega-3s. Other values are for ALA only.

## Best Way to Consume

Fish is one of the best sources of omega-3s for people who are not vegan or vegetarian. It contains highly bioavailable lean protein; omega-3 fatty acids; plus numerous other vitamins, minerals, and zoonutrients (healthful compounds found in animal foods). Because of this synergy of nutrients, it's better to eat fish regularly (two to three times a week at least) than to take supplements.

However, just like not all plant and animal farms are the same, not all fish farms are the same. Fish from sustainable, high-quality fish farms (aquaculture) have no or much lower amounts of mercury, microplastics, and other toxins than most ocean fish. There are also a few certifications to look for when selecting fish. The top ones are the Marine Stewardship Council (MSC), BAP (which certifies aquaculture/farmed fish), and Monterey Bay Aquarium Seafood Watch. A quick look at their websites will give you excellent information on how to choose your seafood.

## Natural Food Sources

| FOOD (SERVING SIZE) | ALA | DHA/EPA |
|---|---|---|
| Trout, farmed from Riverence (3½ ounces) | – | 2.00g |
| Salmon, farmed (3 ounces) | – | 1.24g/0.59g |
| Salmon, wild (1 serving size) | – | 1.22g/0.35g |
| Trout, farmed from McFarland Springs farm (3½ ounces) | – | 0.87g |
| Sardines, canned in tomato sauce, drained (3½ ounces) | – | 0.74g/0.45g |
| Mackerel (3 ounces) | – | 0.59g/0.43g |
| Shrimp, cooked, farmed or wild (3 ounces) | – | 0.12g/0.12g |

| FOOD (SERVING SIZE) | ALA | DHA/EPA |
|---|---|---|
| Flaxseeds, ground (1 tablespoon) | 6.703g | – |
| Hempseed (1 ounce) | 6g | – |
| Chia seeds (1 ounce) | 5.06g | – |
| Walnuts (1 ounce) | 2.57g | – |
| Soybean oil (1 tablespoon) | 0.923g | – |
| Edamame, frozen (½ cup) | 0.28g | – |
| Brussels sprouts, cooked (½ cup) | 0.135g | – |
| Herring, cooked (2 ounces) | 0.05–0.11g | 0.94g/0.77g |
| Tilapia, cooked, farmed or wild (3 ounces) | 0.04g | 0.11g |

## RECIPE

# Steelhead Trout and Curry Vegetables *Serves 2*

I personally recommend the very high-quality, sustainably farmed trout from Riverence. Otherwise, try to make sure you select fish that has been certified from one of the organizations mentioned previously.

1 cup halved Brussels sprouts

1 cup chopped parsnips

1 medium sweet potato, peeled and chopped

2 tablespoons extra-virgin olive oil, divided

⅛ teaspoon salt, divided

⅛ teaspoon black pepper, divided

2 teaspoons curry powder

2 (6-ounce) steelhead trout fillets

2 teaspoons minced garlic

3 teaspoons lemon juice, plus extra for garnish

**PER SERVING**
*Calories: 467,*
*Fat: 24g,*
*Protein: 39g,*
*Sodium: 297mg,*
*Fiber: 6g,*
*Carbohydrates: 22g,*
*Sugar: 4g,*
*Omega-3: 1.9g*

1 Preheat oven to 350°F. Line two baking sheets with aluminum foil.

2 Arrange vegetables evenly on one baking sheet and drizzle with 1 tablespoon olive oil. Toss with pinch salt and pepper, and add in curry powder. Bake 30 minutes or until the sweet potato is soft.

3 Place fish on another baking sheet, and spread garlic and lemon juice evenly over them. Coat with remaining tablespoon oil. Season with remaining salt and pepper. Bake 12–15 minutes.

4 Serve fish drizzled with lemon juice alongside vegetables.

# Omega-6

Omega-6 is a class of fatty acids that is important for your body. There are numerous types of omega-6s, but the main one in our diet is linoleic acid (LA). Our bodies need both omega-3s and omega-6s to function properly and prevent disease, preferring a 1:1 ratio to keep inflammation low. Most people, however, consume fewer omega-3s than omega-6s, with a ratio closer to 20:1 or 30:1 omega-6 to omega-3s! That is a huge imbalance. The vast majority of people need to increase their omega-3s and decrease omega-6s. This could help to lower inflammation and potentially prevent a lot of other health issues.

## Description

Like omega-3s, omega-6s are part of the polyunsaturated fats family. The difference between them is the length of their chemical chains. Linoleic acid has a shorter chain, while arachidonic acid (AA) has a longer chain. The length of these chains affects what they do inside your body. Omega-6s are found in a variety of foods but especially plant oils, specifically corn oil, canola oil, and cottonseed oil.

## Role in the Body

- **Energy:** Fats are essential for energy production and storage.
- **Possibly involved in improved insulin sensitivity:** A large research study published in the medical journal *The Lancet* showed that people with higher blood levels of omega-6, specifically as linoleic acid, had a lower risk of developing diabetes. More research is needed, however, before encouraging increasing omega-6, as the weight of the evidence still indicates that too-high omega-6 intake will increase inflammation.
- **Can help to reduce inflammation when used in place of trans and saturated fats:** The key phrase here is "in place of," not "in addition to." Some research shows that replacing these less healthy fats with omegas can help with inflammation, but we know it's still important to keep a good ratio with omega-3s.
- **Needed for skin and hair growth:** Omega-6s help to form skin and hair cells and keep them healthy.

In addition, another omega-6 fatty acid, conjugated linoleic acid (CLA), is showing promise in some studies with weight management and helping to prevent cancer. CLA is mainly found in grass-fed dairy and meat.

## Benefits

- Proper growth and development
- Normal metabolism
- Healthy skin and hair
- Normal energy levels
- Possibly beneficial for weight management and cancer prevention

Another type of omega-6, gamma linolenic acid (GLA), may potentially help with PMS symptoms and inflammation and pain caused by arthritis. This fatty acid is found in evening primrose oil, borage oil, and black currant seed oil.

## Side Effects, Warnings, and Precautions

If you are like many others who consume too many omega-6s while not eating enough omega-3s, you run the risk of the following:

- Increased risk for heart disease
- Increased risk of cancer
- Higher levels of inflammation
- Higher risk of developing autoimmune conditions

## Signs of Deficiency

Deficiency occurs in people on very low-fat diets or those with problems absorbing fat. Usually, this would show up as a deficiency in all essential fatty acids, not just omega-6.

Signs of deficiency include:

- Fatigue
- Dull or dry skin and hair
- Dermatitis

## How Much You Need (RDA)

| AGE | MALE | FEMALE |
| --- | --- | --- |
| 0–6 months | 4.4g* | 4.4g* |
| 7–12 months | 4.6g* | 4.6g* |
| 1–3 years | 7g | 7g |
| 4–8 years | 10g | 10g |
| 9–13 years | 12g | 10g |
| 14–18 years | 16g | 11g |
| 19–50 years | 17g | 12g |
| 51+ years | 14g | 11g |
| Pregnancy | – | 13g |
| Lactation | – | 13g |

* Amount is estimated from breast milk.

## Best Way to Consume

The best way to consume omega-6 fatty acids in the right amounts is to eat a balance of plant-based foods like nuts, seeds, and oils, while limiting processed foods and those that are particularly high in omega-6. Choose oils like extra-virgin olive oil or avocado oil instead of soy or canola. It is not generally recommended to supplement with omega-6 fatty acids, but in some cases it may be useful to try CLA or GLA supplements for certain conditions; discuss this with your doctor and dietitian.

## Natural Food Sources

| FOOD (SERVING SIZE) | OMEGA-6 (G) |
| --- | --- |
| Corn oil (2 tablespoons) | 14 |
| Soybean oil (2 tablespoons) | 13.8 |
| Firm tofu, cubed (1 cup) | 10.9 |
| Walnuts (2 tablespoons) | 10.6 |
| Sunflower seeds (2 tablespoons) | 9.7 |
| Flaxseed oil (1 tablespoon) | 8.5 |
| Almonds (2 tablespoons) | 3.4 |

## RECIPE

# Anti-Inflammatory Nut and Seed Super Salad *Serves 1*

This salad is packed with healthy fats from the nuts and seeds. You can enjoy this salad with toasted bread or as is and switch up the nuts and seeds to your liking.

1 cup mixed greens

½ cup cooked buckwheat

1 medium tomato, finely chopped

¼ cup crumbled feta cheese

1 tablespoon pine nuts

1 tablespoon pumpkin seeds

1 teaspoon hempseeds

1 tablespoon finely chopped mint

1 tablespoon extra-virgin olive oil

½ tablespoon balsamic vinegar

**PER SERVING**
*Calories: 421, Fat: 28g, Protein: 13g, Sodium: 376mg, Fiber: 6g, Carbohydrates: 29g, Sugar: 7g*

1 Combine all ingredients except oil and vinegar in a large bowl.

2 Dress with oil and vinegar and toss to coat. Enjoy.

# Phosphorus

Phosphorus was accidentally discovered by a German alchemist named Hennig Brand around 1669. He was trying to find the elusive "philosopher's stone," which people at the time thought was a magical substance that would transform metals into gold. Through an arduous process that involved distilling and boiling down urine, he managed to extract nearly pure phosphorus, which glows in the dark. He named it after the Greek word *phosphoros*, which means "bringer of light." Phosphorus is a macro mineral, which means we need more than trace amounts of it in our diet. It is a major component of bones and teeth, along with calcium. Unless you have some type of kidney problem, the chances that your phosphorus levels are out of range are minimal.

## Description

Despite the important role phosphorus plays in your body, you probably don't hear about it very often, because having low or high levels is unusual, and it's also really easy to get plenty of it from the foods you eat. Phosphorus is in almost everything, but especially high-protein foods like meat, dairy, and eggs.

Phosphorus is used by every cell in the body for a few key functions, one of them being energy production. A compound called adenosine triphosphate (ATP) is needed for this energy production and transfer inside of your cells. Phosphate comes from phosphorus, and there are three (tri) molecules of it in ATP.

## Role in the Body

- **Partners up with calcium to build bones and teeth:** 85 percent of the phosphorus in your body is stored in the bones and teeth.
- **Is a key part of energy production in all cells:** As part of ATP, phosphorus helps create the energy that keeps you moving and your metabolism functioning all day long.
- **Is part of DNA and RNA:** Not only is phosphorus needed for energy; it also forms the backbone of the molecules that encode your genetic material: DNA and RNA.
- **Is a component of cell membranes:** Phospholipids, which are fats that contain a phosphate group, help form these key structural components of cells.

## Benefits

- Helps build bones and teeth, along with calcium and vitamin D

- Helps activate numerous signaling molecules like hormones and enzymes
- Protects the integrity of cells and helps form the membranes that keep out invaders like bacteria and viruses
- Acts as a buffer to help the body maintain its proper PH level
- Regulates the delivery of oxygen to all of the body's tissues

## Side Effects, Warnings, and Precautions

Your body has a pretty effective mechanism to keep phosphorus levels in check: If you're not consuming very much, your kidneys will start to absorb more of it from the foods you eat to compensate. People with advanced renal problems, like stage-three or stage-four kidney disease and those on dialysis, should be cautious with their intake and monitor it. The individual amount for these people will vary depending on their laboratory levels. They will need to work with a dietitian to make sure they get a special diet plan that's tailored for them.

One more thing to be aware of is the potential link between too much phosphorus from dark-colored sodas and bone health. More research is needed on the topic, but one large study done by researchers at Tufts University showed that women who drank a high amount of soda (more than three cans per day) had lower bone density and a higher risk of fractures. Dark-colored sodas (like Coke and Pepsi) are much higher in phosphorus than light-colored sodas (like Sprite or 7UP). It isn't totally clear as to why this is the case, but one explanation is if the ratio of calcium and phosphorus in the body gets thrown off, it could be harmful to bone health. If you love soda and find it really tough to give up, aim for just one per day.

## Signs of Deficiency

As mentioned, low phosphorus is very rare, but it does occur in a few specific conditions, such as starvation. Also at risk are alcoholics, people with rare genetic disorders that affect their phosphorus balance, and diabetics with severely out-of-control blood sugars.

Signs of deficiency can include:

- Weakness and fatigue
- Bone pain
- Loss of appetite
- Numbness and tingling
- Increased infections
- Difficulty breathing/respiratory failure

# How Much You Need

| AGE | MALE | FEMALE |
| --- | --- | --- |
| 0–6 months | 100mg | 100mg |
| 7–12 months | 275mg | 275mg |
| 1–3 years | 460mg | 460mg |
| 4–8 years | 500mg | 500mg |
| 9–13 years | 1,250mg | 1,250mg |
| 14–18 years | 1,250mg | 1,250mg |
| 19+ years | 700mg | 700mg |
| Pregnancy and Lactation 18 years and younger | – | 1,250mg |
| Pregnancy and Lactation 19 years and older | – | 700mg |

# Tolerable Upper Intake Levels

| AGE | MALE | FEMALE |
| --- | --- | --- |
| 0–6 months | Not established | Not established |
| 7–12 months | Not established | Not established |
| 1–3 years | 3,000mg | 3,000mg |
| 4–8 years | 3,000mg | 3,000mg |
| 9–13 years | 4,000mg | 4,000mg |
| 14–18 years | 4,000mg | 4,000mg |
| 19–70 years | 4,000mg | 4,000mg |
| 71+ years | 3,000mg | 3,000mg |
| Pregnancy | – | 3,500mg |
| Lactation | – | 4,000mg |

## Best Way to Consume

Nearly all foods have some amount of phosphorous, though some have much more than others. High-protein foods have the most phosphorus—these include animal products like meats, dairy, fish, eggs, and so on. Whole grains and legumes like beans and lentils are also good sources of phosphorus. Fruits and vegetables have little phosphorous. Whether you are vegetarian, vegan, or eat animal products, as long as you're eating a balanced diet and sufficient protein sources, you're almost certainly meeting your phosphorus needs. You'll notice in the AI table that phosphorus needs are highest during adolescence and then decrease after the age of nineteen. Those are the years that bones are forming, and after this period of time you need much less of this mineral.

## Natural Food Sources

| FOOD (SERVING SIZE) | PHOSPHORUS (MG) |
| --- | --- |
| Sardines, canned, drained (3 ounces) | 411 |
| Pumpkin seeds (¼ cup) | 397 |
| Chicken, cooked, meat only (1 cup) | 300 |
| Turkey, cooked, meat only (1 cup) | 300 |
| Milk, skim (1 cup) | 247 |
| Salmon, Atlantic, cooked (3 ounces) | 214 |
| Lentils, cooked (½ cup) | 178 |
| Almonds (23 nuts) | 136 |
| Egg, hard-boiled (1 large) | 86 |
| Bread, whole wheat (1 slice) | 68 |

# Salsa and Lime Chicken Tacos *Serves 1*

Since so many foods have phosphorus, you definitely don't need to make a special recipe to get it, but here's an example of an easy, nutrient-dense meal that also contains this vital mineral and is a healthy spin on a Mexican classic.

---

| | | |
|---|---|---|
| 1 (4-ounce) chicken breast, cut into strips | 1 tablespoon lime juice | 2 corn tortillas |
| 2 ounces salsa | ½ teaspoon chili powder | 1 cup chopped romaine lettuce |

---

**PER SERVING**
*Calories: 243, Fat: 4g, Protein: 29g, Sodium: 146mg, Fiber: 5g, Carbohydrates: 24g, Sugar: 1g, Phosphorus: 387mg*

1 Place chicken strips into a large resealable plastic bag with salsa, lime juice, and chili powder. Allow to marinate at least 1 hour.
2 Heat tortillas in a medium skillet over medium heat, just enough to barely get some brown on each side. Set aside.
3 Add chicken and marinade to the skillet and cook until cooked through, about 8–10 minutes.
4 Serve chicken in tortillas, topped with lettuce.

# Polyphenols

Polyphenols are a category of chemicals that naturally occur in plants. Thousands of different kinds have been discovered, and there are many more that scientists have yet to identify. We've long known that eating more fruits, vegetables, herbs, spices, and other plant foods can improve life span, boost brain health, and reduce the risk for chronic conditions like heart disease, diabetes, and cancer. But what is it specifically about these foods that makes them such an important factor in preventing disease? Research has revealed that an important part of what makes plant foods so beneficial to our health are, you guessed it, polyphenols.

## Description

When you see the bright colors of fruits and vegetables, like the deep purple of a plum or the vibrant green of kale leaves, the compounds that provide these magnificent shades are polyphenols. That luscious flavor of a sweet grape and the complex bitterness of arugula are also provided by polyphenols. The aromatic scent of cocoa and the delicate fragrance of strawberries? Yes, those also come from polyphenols. Many studies and analyses have shown that diets filled with these incredible compounds can help to prevent cancer, heart disease, dementia, and more.

There are four different types of polyphenols, which include:

- **Flavonoids:** This class of polyphenols has been the most studied and includes over five thousand different compounds, many of which give colors to foods and act as antioxidants. Some of the best-known flavonoids are luteolin, quercetin, and catechins.
- **Lignans:** A lesser-studied subgroup of polyphenols, these compounds help to feed the beneficial gut bacteria in your digestive tract and are found in foods like flaxseeds, whole grains, and some fruits and veggies.
- **Stilbenes:** Unlike flavonoids, of which there are thousands, there are only two stilbenes that have been studied in depth: resveratrol and pterostilbene. These are found in foods like wine and peanuts. For example, the health benefits of red wine come from the resveratrol in the grape skins.
- **Phenolic acids:** These compounds are known to have strong anti-inflammatory and antioxidant actions. The highest concentrations are found in the skins and seeds of fruits and leaves of vegetables. Some foods

known for their antioxidant benefits thanks to phenolic acids are coffee, tea, cherries, kiwis, and some whole-grain flours like corn, wheat, and oat.

Gut health is yet another area where polyphenols play a beneficial role. The good bugs in your gut need something to eat, and that is often in the form of polyphenols. Polyphenols not only help to support the good bacteria in your body; they also help to diversify them. People with more varied strains and higher numbers of the good bugs tend to have better health outcomes.

## Role in the Body

- **Weight management:** Some research has shown that eating polyphenols can help people to maintain a healthy weight and waist circumference.
- **Gut bacteria:** Polyphenols support the "good bugs" and help keep your digestive system healthy.
- **Preventing neurodegeneration:** Polyphenols may increase blood flow to the brain, thus helping it to detox from wastes and maintain normal function.
- **Blood sugar regulation:** Certain types of polyphenols found in spices like rosemary, ginger, oregano, and black pepper as well as in dark chocolate, tofu, and pomegranates can help

improve how your body processes sugar and carbs.

- **Blood pressure modulation:** Some studies have evaluated how polyphenols in cocoa can affect heart health. Research has shown that eating cocoa for a period of only two weeks decreased blood pressure significantly in study participants.
- **Antioxidant activity:** One of the main benefits of polyphenols is their ability to neutralize harmful compounds called free radicals.
- **Skin protection:** Due to their ability to fight off free radicals, polyphenols help protect the skin from aging.
- **Anti-inflammatory activity:** Chronic inflammation can wreak havoc on your system by increasing stress hormones and leading to disease. Polyphenols help to minimize and reduce some of this response naturally.

## Benefits

- **Reduced risk of stroke:** By helping to decrease blood pressure, polyphenols decrease the risk of hypertension and stroke.
- **Lower risk of type 2 diabetes:** By helping your body process sugars and respond to insulin, polyphenols reduce the risk of this chronic condition.
- **Younger-looking skin:** The antioxidant power of polyphenols helps to

keep your skin looking youthful and healthy.

- **May protect from diseases like Parkinson's and Alzheimer's:** Flavonoids' anti-inflammatory and antioxidant effects may help protect against neurodegenerative diseases like Alzheimer's and Parkinson's.
- **Heart health:** Polyphenols can reduce the risk for heart disease by lowering buildup of bad cholesterol and possibly improving the health of blood vessels.
- **Antiaging:** By reducing inflammation and combatting harmful free radicals, polyphenols can act as natural antiaging compounds.
- **Improved digestion:** The microbiome requires all kinds of nutrients to thrive, and polyphenols can help boost its health by supporting the good gut bacteria.
- **Weight loss:** Studies have uncovered a link between upregulation of an appetite-suppressing hormone naturally made in our bodies, leptin, and some flavonoids, meaning that getting more flavonoids could help reduce cravings and appetite and help with weight management.
- **Stronger immune system:** One of the reasons plants have polyphenols is to help fight off disease and invaders. When you consume them, your immune system is also strengthened.

## Side Effects, Warnings, and Precautions

There are few risks from consuming polyphenols from food sources. Supplements that contain higher doses of polyphenols may cause side effects, and since they are concentrated they may contain higher levels of environmental contaminants as well. Some high-dose quercetin supplements, for example, have caused nausea and vomiting. There's also a chance that some foods with polyphenols can affect the absorption of certain other nutrients and vitamins from foods, and could interact with medications. For example, the polyphenols in grapefruit juice can potentiate the effects of certain medications like painkillers and calcium channel blockers.

## Signs of Deficiency

Polyphenols are not (yet) considered an essential food, but there are definitely risks to not consuming enough of them. People who don't eat enough plant-based foods are probably low in their polyphenol intake.

Signs of deficiency can include:

- Accelerated aging of the skin and sun damage
- Weight gain
- Fatigue and sluggishness

## How Much You Need

There isn't a set Daily Value (a percentage guide on the Nutrition Facts label as to the nutrients in a serving) at this time for these compounds, but following the guidelines for fruit and vegetable intake as well as legumes, such as peanuts, is an excellent place to start. The current guidelines recommend five servings of fruits and vegetables per day. You can also try adding herbs and spices like rosemary, dill, or basil to your meals in place of salt. That way you reduce sodium (which most people eat too much of) and boost polyphenols (which most people are deficient in) while adding lots of variety and flavor to your meals.

## Best Way to Consume

Simply adding an additional cup of fresh or frozen fruits and vegetables to your diet each day is an effective way to boost your polyphenols. Consuming them as fresh as possible and not cutting them up until you are ready to eat them will preserve more of the nutrients. Research has shown that these compounds tend to be more concentrated in and close to the outer skin, so leaving the skin on (when it's edible) is ideal.

Choose organic whenever possible, and eat the skins of foods like apples, pears, cucumbers, and sweet potatoes. Add spices to your dishes. A sprinkle of cinnamon on your cereal or some cacao nibs on top of your oatmeal are simple and delicious options. Snacking on nuts and seeds is also a great way to get polyphenols. For example, roasted (unsalted) peanuts have a high amount of a polyphenol called p-coumaric acid, which has strong antioxidant effects.

## Natural Food Sources

There are innumerable sources of polyphenols. You can get them from eating almost any plant-based food! *The European Journal of Clinical Nutrition* published a list of the one hundred richest dietary sources of polyphenols, based on milligrams per 100 grams. Here are the twenty foods that topped that list:

**FOOD SOURCES**

| | |
|---|---|
| Cloves | Dried sage |
| Peppermint | Spearmint |
| Star anise | Rosemary |
| Raw cacao | Thyme |
| Mexican oregano | Blueberries |
| Celery seeds | Black currants |
| Dark chocolate | Capers |
| Flaxseed meal | Black olives |
| Black elderberries | Hazelnuts |
| Chestnut seeds | Pecans |

## OTHER FOOD SOURCES—FRUITS, VEGETABLES, NUTS, SEEDS

| | |
|---|---|
| Prunes | Plums |
| Potatoes | Green olives |
| Curry powder | Sweet cherries |
| Globe artichoke heads | Ginger, dried |
| Broccoli | Black tea |
| Green tea | Soy yogurt |
| Strawberries | Blackgrapes |
| Yellow onions | Black beans |
| Pure pomegranate juice | Pure blood orange juice |
| Apricots | Walnuts |

## RECIPE

# Cherry Chocolate Peanut Polyphenol Boost Bowl *Serves 1*

This superfood bowl is a great way to start the day feeling refreshed. Packed with polyphenols and flavor it will help your digestion and improve your skin health.

½ medium frozen banana, peeled

½ cup frozen acai

½ cup frozen berries

½ cup coconut water

1 teaspoon ground cinnamon

1 tablespoon cacao nibs

1 tablespoon unsalted peanut butter, melted

2 tablespoons dried cherries

**PER SERVING**
*Calories: 364, Fat: 15g, Protein: 7g, Sodium: 137mg, Fiber: 15g, Carbohydrates: 54g, Sugar: 30g*

1 In a blender, mix banana, acai, berries, coconut water, and cinnamon.

2 Transfer to a small bowl and top with cacao nibs, a drizzle of peanut butter, and cherries. Enjoy!

# Potassium

Potassium is a mineral that is present in every cell in the body. It can help lower your blood pressure, protect your muscles, preserve your bones, and so much more. It should be easy to get plenty of potassium because it's in so many different foods, but recent dietary surveys show that in fact, many people don't get enough. The Dietary Guidelines for Americans called potassium a "nutrient of concern" because so many Americans don't consume sufficient amounts. Keep reading to find out the best ways to get more potassium into your diet.

## Description

Let's cut to the chase: You probably need more potassium. Since it is mostly found in fruits and vegetables, starting out your day with these foods and trying to include them with each meal is the easiest way to boost your potassium intake.

Potassium is one of the minerals that is also an electrolyte (as are sodium and chloride). Electrolytes transmit electrical nerve signals in your body. Because of this function, potassium is essential for proper functioning of your heart, kidneys, and muscles. Research has also shown many links between potassium and blood pressure. While the exact mechanisms of this connection are not fully understood, it seems that consuming extra potassium can help to offset the negative effects of sodium on blood pressure, thus reducing it, as well as reducing the risk for heart disease and stroke.

## Role in the Body

- **One of the main electrolytes in the body:** Potassium works mostly inside of your cells to maintain proper fluid balance, which helps you feel hydrated and healthy.
- **Keeps your heart and muscles firing properly:** As the key electrolyte inside your cells, potassium helps transmit signals to keep your heartbeat steady and your muscles moving.
- **Helps to flush out excess sodium in the body:** When you eat too much salt, potassium will help to balance it out and flush some of the excess out of your system.
- **Nerve impulse transmission:** Potassium conducts electrical charges to keep the communication channels between the brain and body working correctly.

## Benefits

- **Helps keep blood pressure at a healthy level:** Potassium balances fluids and helps get rid of extra salt (sodium) if there's too much of it.
- **Reduces water retention and bloating:** By flushing out excess salt and fluids, potassium can help release excess water and reduce bloating and swelling.
- **May help to prevent osteoporosis (weakening of the bones):** Potassium reduces the amount of calcium lost through the urine. Some studies have shown that women with high potassium intakes have stronger bones.
- **Prevents kidney stones:** By reducing calcium in the urine, potassium helps prevent the formation of painful kidney stones.
- **May help to lower blood sugar:** People with low intakes of potassium seem to have higher blood sugar levels, which can lead to diabetes over time.
- **May help to prevent strokes and heart disease:** Some studies have shown that people who eat a potassium-rich diet have much lower rates of strokes and heart disease compared to those who don't.

## Side Effects, Warnings, and Precautions

Getting too much of this mineral from foods is almost impossible. However, potassium supplements can sometimes provide too much potassium and are usually unnecessary. Unless there's a medically mandated reason for supplements, it's ideal to get all of your potassium from foods.

The kidneys work to balance out the potassium levels in the blood, so people with kidney problems need to monitor their intake. Additionally, some heart medications can interact with potassium and cause the amount to become elevated. These include ACE inhibitors and diuretics. Make sure to check with your doctor if you have any heart or kidney issues to get personalized recommendations for your needs.

## Signs of Deficiency

It's rare to see actual potassium deficiency, but a large number of people have suboptimal intakes because they don't eat enough potassium-rich foods.

Also, people with certain conditions or those on some medications may be at higher risk for lower potassium levels, including:

- Those with gastrointestinal disorders that affect their absorption of nutrients and ability to eat certain foods (like those diagnosed with inflammatory bowel disease conditions) may have lower potassium levels.

- People who take laxatives over a long period of time as well as certain types of diuretics may be at risk.
- Anyone losing a lot of fluids from diarrhea, vomiting, and heavy sweating may see a drop in their potassium and other electrolyte levels (this is why it's important to replenish large fluid losses with an electrolyte solution and not just plain water).
- People with kidney failure and on dialysis are at high risk for potassium fluctuations.

Signs of deficiency can include:

- Constipation
- Weakness/tiredness
- Elevated blood pressure
- Increased urination
- High blood sugar
- Increased risk of kidney stones
- Irregular heartbeat

**How Much You Need**
There is no RDA or upper limit for potassium. The following table shows Adequate Intake amounts.

| AGE | MALE | FEMALE |
|---|---|---|
| 0–6 months | 400mg | 400mg |
| 7–12 months | 860mg | 860mg |
| 1–3 years | 2,000mg | 2,000mg |
| 4–8 years | 2,300mg | 2,300mg |
| 9–13 years | 2,500mg | 2,300mg |
| 14–18 years | 3,000mg | 2,300mg |
| 19–50 years | 3,400mg | 2,600mg |
| 51+ years | 3,400mg | 2,600mg |
| Pregnancy | – | 2,900mg |
| Lactation | – | 2,800mg |

## Best Way to Consume

Since fruits and vegetables are the foods highest in this key nutrient, you should start eating them early in the day. It can be tough to get all the servings you need (the official recommendation is about five to seven, though you should try to aim for ten if possible) if you only begin eating fruits and vegetables in the afternoon. Fresh smoothies are a delicious and easy way to get your fruit and vegetable servings plus many other key nutrients.

## Natural Food Sources

| FOOD (SERVING SIZE) | POTASSIUM (MG) |
| --- | --- |
| Apricots, dried (½ cup) | 1,101 |
| Lentils, cooked (1 cup) | 731 |
| Prunes, dried (½ cup) | 699 |
| Yam, baked (3½ ounces) | 670 |
| Beet greens, cooked (½ cup) | 654 |
| Squash, acorn, peeled, mashed (1 cup) | 644 |
| Pomegranate juice (1 cup) | 533 |
| Avocado (3½ ounces or 7 tablespoons) | 485 |
| Edamame beans (3½ ounces) | 436 |
| Banana, peeled (1 medium) | 422 |
| Peaches, pitted, sliced (¼ cup) | 399 |
| Spinach, raw (2 cups) | 334 |
| Asparagus, cooked, chopped (½ cup) | 202 |
| Brown rice (1 cup) | 154 |

# Tropical Morning Smoothie *Serves 1*

This morning recipe will help you balance electrolyte levels in your body. Smoothies are a great way to pack in nutrients while staying hydrated.

1 cup baby kale

½ cup coconut water

½ medium frozen banana, peeled

¼ cup frozen pineapple chunks

½ medium orange, peeled and sliced

2 tablespoons chia seeds

Ice, as desired

**PER SERVING**
*Calories: 230, Fat: 6g, Protein: 6g, Sodium: 135mg, Fiber: 13g, Carbohydrates: 41g, Sugar: 21g, Potassium: 833mg*

Add all ingredients to a blender and mix until smooth. Enjoy!

# Sweet and Savory Salad *Serves 1*

Since potassium is so important, I'm providing two recipes here: one for the afternoon and one for the morning. This sweet and savory salad has a perfectly balanced flavor. It's rich in potassium plus many other essential nutrients. Make more to pack for lunch!

2 cups watercress

¼ cup baked sweet potato cubes

½ cup cooked lentils

¼ cup chopped dried apricots

¼ medium avocado, peeled, pitted, and sliced

1 tablespoon pomegranate seeds

1 tablespoon chopped fresh mint

Pinch salt

Pinch black pepper

1 tablespoon extra-virgin olive oil

**PER SERVING**
*Calories: 428, Fat: 18g, Protein: 13g, Sodium: 341mg, Fiber: 15g, Carbohydrates: 57g, Sugar: 24g, Potassium: 1,403mg*

1 Add all ingredients except oil into a medium bowl.
2 Drizzle with oil and mix well. Enjoy!

# Prebiotics

You may have heard of probiotics, but have you heard of their equally important but lesser-known counterpart, prebiotics? The prefix "pro-" means "for" (so "probiotics" means "for life"). The prefix "pre-" indicates that something has to come "before." Thus, prebiotics are an essential piece of the gut health and microbiota puzzle, helping to encourage the growth of probiotics, the beneficial bacteria in your digestive tract. You can think of prebiotics as the foods that feed probiotics. Prebiotics are mostly found in fruits, vegetables, nuts, seeds, and whole grains as fiber. People who don't eat enough of these nutrient-dense foods are also lacking in prebiotics.

## Description

The term "you are what you eat" has never been more true. We now know that the foods we eat directly influence the types of bacteria that grow inside of our guts, also termed the microbiota. The microbiota refers to the trillions of bacterial cells as well as viruses, parasites, and fungi inside each of us, mostly found in the digestive tract. Until relatively recently, the microbiota's role in our health was not as well appreciated as it is now. Globally, there are many research projects underway to better understand the complex and fascinating contributions the microbiota provides and its implications for our health.

Prebiotics are essential for supporting the microbiota. They are typically carbs that your body can't fully digest but that are instead used by the bacteria in your intestines. There are many different kinds of prebiotics, but some of the most well studied include inulin, oligosaccharides, and polydextrose. That's a mouthful, but don't worry, you don't need to remember these names; what's most important is to focus on increasing the foods that are high in prebiotics, which you can easily do by increasing your complex carb consumption.

Prebiotics have some fascinating functions. For example, they may play an important role in the prevention of allergies. They also can have a positive immune effect in the gut as a result of fermentation, which creates short-chain fatty acids (SCFAs). These SCFAs in turn have a direct anti-inflammatory effect and may help improve the integrity of the intestinal wall.

Recent research has shown that a diet higher in plant-based foods (i.e., prebiotics) promotes much greater diversity among the various strains of gut bacteria inside your body. People who consume higher amounts of meat and not enough vegetables tend to have less diversity in the strains that colonize their guts. Dairy products seem to help with a variety of bacteria as well. Even geography seems to make a difference; one research study showed that people who live in developing nations have a greater diversity in their microbiota than people who live in developed nations.

## Role in the Body

- **Stimulate growth of healthy bacteria:** Prebiotics are like fertilizer for the microbiota. When you're planting a garden, you need to nourish the soil the plants grow in—if they have the right amounts of nutrition, they will burst into bloom.
- **Promote intestinal integrity:** Prebiotics promote the growth of certain types of bacteria that improve the intestinal wall barrier.
- **Anti-inflammatory:** By supporting the formation of SCFA and providing a protective effect in the intestinal lining, prebiotics help to reduce inflammation.
- **May improve immune function:** When the gut is healthy and the intestinal tract is intact, your immune system is optimized.
- **May improve absorption of calcium and magnesium:** By improving the integrity of the intestinal wall, there is an increase in the surface area of the intestines, which allows for greater absorption of minerals.

## Benefits

- Improved digestion
- May improve bone health
- May lower stress response
- Improved hormonal balance
- Lowered risk of weight gain
- Decreased risk of developing allergies

## Side Effects, Warnings, and Precautions

Some types of prebiotics can be aggravating to those with GI issues, especially conditions like small intestinal bacterial overgrowth (SIBO), irritable bowel syndrome (IBS), and Crohn's disease. People who have GI issues should check with their doctor and dietitian before increasing their prebiotic intake.

There is also a potential for acid reflux when adding extra prebiotics to your diet. You should take it slow and add them gradually if you are prone to acid reflux issues.

Adding a lot of prebiotics at once can actually cause distress to your system because of the fibrous content, so go slow and introduce them gradually, over a few weeks.

## Signs of Deficiency

People with gastrointestinal disorders, absorption disorders, and those who can't tolerate high amounts of fiber can potentially become deficient in prebiotics.

Signs of deficiency can include:

- Diarrhea
- Constipation
- Inflammation
- Greater susceptibility to infections
- Possible weight gain

## How Much You Need

There is currently no established RDA for prebiotics. More research is needed to establish the levels of these nutrients that are necessary, safe, and efficacious for human health. Because most prebiotic foods are high in fiber, you can follow the fiber recommendations (approximately 25–40 grams per day) to ensure you're getting enough.

## Best Way to Consume

The best way to increase your intake of prebiotics is to take in more fresh fruits and vegetables and to select whole grains (like whole-wheat bread) instead of processed grains (like white bread).

Natural foods with high prebiotic components are noted in the following list. It's also very important to drink extra water when increasing your intake of prebiotics, and to increase your intake gradually. Suddenly eating a lot of fiber if your system isn't used to it can cause unpleasant side effects, like gas, bloating, and constipation. Add one or two prebiotic foods every couple of days and build from there.

## Natural Food Sources

- Chicory root
- Asparagus
- Garlic
- Onion
- Bananas
- Jerusalem artichoke
- Oats
- Apples
- Cocoa
- Soybeans
- Leeks
- Whole wheat
- Flaxseed
- Jicama roots
- Seaweed
- Dandelion greens

**RECIPE**

# Chocolate Pecan Prebiotic Smoothie *Serves 1*

Enjoy this treat as a smoothie or smoothie bowl topped with your choice of fresh fruit, nuts, and seeds.

½ medium frozen banana, peeled

½ cup blueberries (frozen for thicker consistency)

¾ cup almond milk

2 tablespoons pecan halves

2 teaspoons raw cocoa powder

1 teaspoon chicory root powder

1 teaspoon flaxseeds

Ice, as needed

**PER SERVING**
*Calories: 262, Fat: 9g, Protein: 6g, Sodium: 114mg, Fiber: 12g, Carbohydrates: 35g, Sugar: 22g*

1  Add all ingredients, except ice, to a blender and mix well.

2  Add ice cubes as desired to adjust consistency.

# Probiotics

The word "probiotics" was invented in 1965 to signify something that is the opposite of antibiotics, which obliterate bacteria. Thus, probiotics means something that is "for life" or that promotes the growth of beneficial bacteria and other substances like some yeasts. Most of these healthful organisms in your body reside in your digestive tract. The significance of the gut in your overall well-being cannot be overstated. For example, we now know that 90 percent of serotonin in the body (the chemical that helps you feel happy) is made in the gut. If your digestive system is out of balance, it can affect almost everything else, including mood, energy levels, joint health, and immunity (in fact, most of your immune function is in your intestinal tract). As more evidence emerges on the tremendous role your gut plays in your overall health, it's becoming more and more clear that keeping this delicate ecosystem of gut bugs and cells flourishing is essential to your physical and mental well-being.

## Description

Long before the word "probiotic" existed, many societies knew about the benefits of probiotic-rich foods. Fermentation, a process of food preservation, has been used for millennia by different societies. Kimchi in Korean cuisine, natto and miso in Japanese dishes, and the list goes on and on. Eating a more processed diet puts you at risk for missing out on these superfoods.

Another factor to keep in mind is that probiotics don't just survive and thrive on their own. They also need sources of nourishment. These sources are called *pre*biotics (see the previous entry on prebiotics). But in short, the best foods to nourish your gut flora are plant-based and full of fiber. Think leafy greens, nuts, seeds, herbs, and whole grains.

## Role in the Body

- **Digestion of foods:** Probiotics feed on fibers and help to break them down so they can pass through your system more efficiently.
- **Immune health:** 70 percent of the body's immune system is in the intestinal tract, so keeping it populated with the good bugs helps you stay healthy and fight off bad invaders.
- **Balance of pH levels in the gut:** Some probiotics help produce compounds that combat unhealthy pH levels and restore balance.
- **Absorption of nutrients:** By digesting certain nutrients and making

them more bioavailable to the body, probiotics help you absorb macro- and micronutrients.

- **Suppression of inflammation:** By producing special types of fatty acids that reduce the inflammatory response, probiotics help prevent chronic inflammation.
- **Production of nutrients:** Some probiotics have the amazing ability to biosynthesize (create) vitamins, which include vitamin K and many of the B vitamins.
- **Heart health:** By breaking down bile, certain types of bacteria can help reduce buildup of unhealthy fats in the body.

## Benefits

- Smooth breakdown and processing of what you eat so that it's well absorbed
- Protect the body from pathogens and invaders that cause illness
- Alleviate constipation, gas, and bloating
- Reduce diarrhea from different causes and restore normal stools
- Can reduce symptoms of lactose intolerance
- May have links to cancer reduction
- May reduce blood pressure
- Can reduce cholesterol
- May help with blood sugar balance

- Prevent yeast infections
- May help with mood disorders such as depression and anxiety
- May reduce the risk of obesity

## Side Effects, Warnings, and Precautions

Probiotics sometimes sound like a miracle product that can cure all of your ills, depending on what source you listen to or read. While they are undoubtedly important, even essential, to good health, there are many claims by manufacturers that want to capitalize on the growing public interest in probiotics that are not necessarily substantiated by research. Be cautious of claims that sound too good to be true, especially from companies looking to sell expensive supplements. As with other supplements, there is little oversight and regulation of the quality, purity, and validity of these products. If you're not able to meet your needs from food sources, check out reliable sources and third-party testing such as Consumer Reports and ConsumerLab.com for information on brands and claims before dropping a lot of money on products that may not deliver on their promises.

Additionally, people who are sick or elderly, or who have weakened immune systems, should not take probiotics without discussing it with their doctor, as potentially dangerous side effects and infections may occur.

## Signs of Deficiency

Individuals who don't consume probiotic-rich foods are at risk of having inadequate probiotic status. Also, people who have absorption disorders and can't tolerate high-fiber foods or other probiotic-rich foods like dairy may have a hard time getting enough probiotics as well as supporting adequate growth of bacterial colonies.

Signs of deficiency can include:

- Mood disorders
- Yeast infections
- High lipid levels
- Weakened immune function
- Fatigue/low energy
- Gastrointestinal problems such as bloating, gas, constipation, and diarrhea
- Weight fluctuations/weight gain

## How Much You Need

There's no set Recommended Daily Allowance (RDA) at this time for probiotics because there isn't enough research on how much is needed for optimal health. There are many differences between individuals as well, so it's difficult to make broad or generalized recommendations. It's a good idea to meet with a registered dietitian to discuss your personalized needs and how to incorporate sufficient amounts of probiotic-rich foods into your diet.

## Best Way to Consume

Ideally, you should be eating something with probiotics every day. It's a great idea to get lots of variety so that you can ensure you're diversifying your gut flora as much as possible. Eating a variety of plant-based foods to help the probiotics in your body thrive is essential as well. As with most nutrients, getting them from foods is ideal. Supplements can be very expensive, and the quality and quantity of probiotics they provide vary drastically. Numerous studies have shown that many probiotic supplements are ineffective, with many of the colonies of organisms being destroyed by the powerful acid in our stomachs before they even make it to the gut, or not being well absorbed. Another recent study showed that even when taking the same type of probiotic, different people will have different absorption and uptake rates. Optimizing your prebiotic intake and eating foods that contain probiotics is a more effective way to improve your gut health.

## Natural Food Sources

Some labels list the number of CFUs (colony-forming units) present in a food. Here are some examples of great sources of probiotics. Generally, higher amounts are more effective.

| FOOD | NUTRIENT (CFU) (THIS WILL VARY DEPENDING ON BRAND AND FORMULATION. THESE NUMBERS ARE ONLY ESTIMATES.) |
| --- | --- |
| Yogurt | $240 \times 10^6$ |
| Kefir | $10^8$ |
| Sauerkraut | $3 \times 10^6$ |
| Kimchi | $10^7 - 10^9$ |
| Miso | $10^{5.8} - 10^{7.4}$ |
| Kombucha | $10^{6.6} - 10^{7.4}$ |
| Sourdough bread | $10^8$ |

Some additional sources of probiotic foods include:

- Apple cider vinegar
- Buttermilk
- Cultured cottage cheese
- Dill pickles (check the label, as not all types have probiotics)
- Garlic
- Kvass (fermented Russian /Ukrainian beverage made from bread)
- Natto
- Olives
- Soft cheeses like Gouda that are made with cultures
- Tempeh (fermented soy)

## RECIPE

# Perfect Probiotic Breakfast Bowl *Serves 1*

Here's a yummy recipe that is symbiotic, meaning it provides both prebiotics (food for probiotics) and probiotic strains to optimize your gut health and good bug balance. Drizzle with a little bit of your favorite sweetener, like agave or honey, if you'd like.

| | | |
| --- | --- | --- |
| 1 (5-ounce) container low-fat, plain Greek yogurt | ½ medium pear, peeled, cored, and sliced<br>½ cup raspberries | 1 tablespoon flaxseed<br>2 tablespoons low-sugar granola |

**PER SERVING**

*Calories: 295, Fat: 8g, Protein: 19g, Sodium: 77mg, Fiber: 11g, Carbohydrates: 39g, Sugar: 19g*

Add yogurt to a small bowl and top with the rest of the ingredients.

# Selenium

The word "selenium" has its roots in Greek mythology: It was named for Selene, the goddess of the moon. Swedish scientist Jöns Jacob Berzelius discovered selenium in 1817 during an analysis of a reddish substance that was contaminating the sulfuric acid being made at a factory. He realized it was a mineral that had not yet been identified. It took many more years to realize what a valuable role selenium plays inside and outside of the body. Today, in addition to the biological functions this trace mineral has, it's also used in solar cells and anti-dandruff products. But in terms of your body, selenium is essential for healthy thyroid function, helps the immune system, and is even linked to cancer and heart disease prevention. While selenium is mainly found in animal products, there's one vegan superfood that contains an entire day's worth of selenium in just one tiny serving—the Brazil nut!

## Description

Despite the fact that you only need selenium in very small amounts, its effect on the body is mighty. Selenium works in synergy with vitamin E to help protect cells from oxidative damage, and is needed for a healthy thyroid gland and your immune system. You require selenium for many metabolic activities and enzymes, including ones that affect reproduction. There's still much research to be done on the various functions and effects of selenium, but some of the active areas that scientists are evaluating include its potential to prevent and treat conditions like heart disease, dementia, cancer, and thyroid conditions.

## Role in the Body

- **Thyroid function:** Most of the selenium in the body is stored in the thyroid gland, which regulates your metabolism and body temperature. Selenium helps to make some of the thyroid hormones that keep this crucial organ functioning properly.
- **Antioxidant capacity:** This mineral is a powerful antioxidant and helps block one of the main pathways responsible for inflammation.
- **DNA repair:** Selenium is needed to support the mechanisms that fix your genes and protect them from damage.
- **Boosts your defense mechanisms:** Also important for immune function, selenium helps your system stay healthy and be less susceptible to both chronic and acute illnesses.

## Benefits

- Helps to prevent hypothyroidism and other thyroid conditions, especially in women
- May help prevent cancer (gastrointestinal, colon, lung, and breast cancers in particular)
- May lower risk of Alzheimer's and other degenerative conditions
- Lowers the risk of heart disease
- Helps strengthen the immune system

## Side Effects, Warnings, and Precautions

The optimal range for selenium is pretty narrow. Getting too much can be toxic and in extreme cases, even fatal. It's unusual to get excess selenium from just food sources (unless you're eating too many Brazil nuts!), but you can definitely get too much from supplements. You should avoid selenium supplements unless there's a medically indicated reason to take them.

Early signs of excessive selenium intake include garlicky breath and a metallic taste in the mouth. If high levels become more severe, hair and nail loss, dizziness, nausea, and vomiting are some of the symptoms. Too much selenium may also affect blood sugar levels and has been correlated with diabetes and poor glucose (blood sugar) control. Anyone who is diabetic should avoid selenium supplements, and if you have other conditions or take other medications, check with your doctor before starting this supplement, as there can be interactions.

## Signs of Deficiency

Selenium deficiency is not seen much in the US and Canada. However, there are deficiencies in some regions, like parts of China and Russia, especially where soil selenium levels are very low and the main diet is vegetarian. Other conditions that have been linked with selenium deficiency are HIV and being on kidney dialysis.

Signs of deficiency can include:

- Brain fog
- Fatigue and weakness
- Hair loss
- Increased infections
- Issues with fertility in both men and women

## How Much You Need (RDA)

| AGE | MALE | FEMALE |
| --- | --- | --- |
| 0–6 months | 15mcg (AI) | 15mcg (AI) |
| 7–12 months | 20mcg (AI) | 20mcg (AI) |
| 1–3 years | 20mcg | 20mcg |
| 4–8 years | 30mcg | 30mcg |
| 9–13 years | 40mcg | 40mcg |
| 14–18 years | 55mcg | 55mcg |

| AGE | MALE | FEMALE |
|---|---|---|
| 19–50 years | 55mcg | 55mcg |
| 51+ years | 55mcg | 55mcg |
| Pregnancy | – | 60mcg |
| Lactation | – | 70mcg |

## Upper Limit (Amount Per Day)

| AGE | MALE | FEMALE |
|---|---|---|
| 0–6 months | 45mcg | 45mcg |
| 7–12 months | 60mcg | 60mcg |
| 1–3 years | 90mcg | 90mcg |
| 4–8 years | 150mcg | 150mcg |
| 9–13 years | 280mcg | 280mcg |
| 14–18 years | 400mcg | 400mcg |
| 19+ years | 400mcg | 400mcg |

| AGE | MALE | FEMALE |
|---|---|---|
| Pregnancy | – | 400mcg |
| Lactation | – | 400mcg |

## Best Way to Consume

One Brazil nut a day keeps selenium deficiency at bay! These creamy and yummy nuts are truly a superfood and often contain more selenium than any other source, in addition to some healthy fats and fiber. The actual content varies depending on the soil they are grown in, but they usually have high amounts of the mineral. Of course, many animal products are good sources of selenium as well, which is where most people get the majority of their selenium intake. These include organ meats like liver, seafood such as fish and shrimp, and chicken.

## Natural Food Sources

| FOOD (SERVING SIZE) | SELENIUM (MCG) |
|---|---|
| Brazil nuts (1 ounce) | 544 |
| Tuna, yellow fin, cooked, dry heat (3 ounces) | 92 |
| Shrimp, canned (3 ounces) | 40 |
| Beef liver, pan fried (3 ounces) | 28 |
| Chicken, light meat, roasted (3 ounces) | 22 |
| Cottage cheese, 1% milk fat (1 cup) | 20 |
| Brown rice, cooked (1 cup) | 19 |
| Egg, hard-boiled (1 large) | 15 |
| Oatmeal, regular or quick, cooked with water (1 cup) | 13 |
| Spinach, cooked from frozen (1 cup) | 11 |

# Pasta with Brazil Nut Pesto *Serves 2*

Pesto is an Italian classic. Make it an excellent source of selenium by adding Brazil nuts. The unique flavor of Brazil nuts makes this dish extra delicious. Serve with whole-wheat pasta for extra fiber.

---

1 clove garlic

4 Brazil nuts

½ cup spinach

½ cup fresh basil

2 tablespoons extra-virgin olive oil, plus more if needed

Juice of ½ medium lemon

Pinch salt

Pinch black pepper

1½ cups cooked whole-wheat pasta

¼ cup grated Parmesan cheese, for garnish

---

**PER SERVING**

*Calories: 378, Fat: 24g, Protein: 12g, Sodium: 812mg, Fiber: 6g, Carbohydrates: 31g, Sugar: 1g, Selenium: 196mcg*

1  In a blender or food processor, add garlic, Brazil nuts, spinach, basil, oil, lemon juice, salt, and pepper and blend until consistency is smooth.

2  If a smoother consistency is needed, add more oil.

3  Serve on top of whole-wheat pasta sprinkled with Parmesan cheese.

# Sodium

When you think of major public health hazards, what comes to mind? Not wearing seat belts? Smoking? Pollution? What about salt? It's in many of the foods we eat and is one of the major threats to our health—causing more deaths annually than car accidents. Research published in *The New England Journal of Medicine* indicates that 1.65 million deaths worldwide each year are directly attributable to eating too much salt. So how did we get to this point and what can be done? Let's find out.

## Description

Salt tastes really good, and it's really cheap (this is why many food manufacturers add it to products—it makes almost anything taste better). During Paleolithic times, when many humans were hunter-gatherers, sodium intake was very low (since processed foods didn't exist!), and some theorize that we may have evolved to desire it, because it *is* an essential nutrient that our body requires to function properly. Today, however, nearly everyone consumes more than they need. If you want to decrease your salt intake, the easiest way is to eat less processed (manufactured/packaged) food and eat at restaurants and fast-food chains less frequently. The other thing you can do to help minimize the impact of salt on your health is increase how much potassium, calcium, and magnesium you eat. These nutrients can actually counteract the negative effects of salt and lower blood pressure. The best way to get more of them is to eat more fruits, vegetables, and other plant-based foods like nuts, seeds, and legumes. Lower-fat dairy and certain fish like sardines are also good sources of calcium.

## Role in the Body

Sodium isn't all bad; it has many essential functions in the body, such as:

- **Nerve impulse transmission:** As one of the electrolyte minerals, sodium helps nerve signals move throughout the body.
- **Regulation of blood pressure:** While too much sodium increases blood pressure, our bodies need just the right amount to keep it stable and at a healthy level.
- **Muscle relaxation:** Sodium assists your muscles, such as the heart, in relaxing.
- **Balance of fluids:** Sodium helps control the amount of fluids inside and outside your cells to ensure homeostasis (balance).

## Benefits

- Helps your muscles contract and relax
- Ensures that your heart beats properly
- Generates electricity to keep your nerves firing
- Maintains fluid balance so you feel hydrated and healthy
- Keeps blood pressure constant when consumed in the right amounts

## Side Effects, Warnings, and Precautions

Interestingly, about one in four people is "salt sensitive," according to the American Heart Association. This means their body responds even more to sodium because they are genetically predisposed to be extra sensitive to salt. Their blood pressure will rise higher than the average person with additional intake, and this will cause negative effects even sooner. Nutrigenomic testing, which looks at genetic variations in nutrition markers, can tell you if you are in this group. However, you can still decrease the amount you eat even without a nutrigenomics test.

Too much salt can cause the following negative effects:

- Fluid retention, swelling, and bloating
- Calcium losses, which will weaken bones
- High blood pressure (hypertension)

- Heart disease
- Stroke
- Kidney damage
- Increased risk of stomach cancer

## Signs of Deficiency

Some rare genetic conditions can cause low sodium, such as Addison's disease and Bartter syndrome. People who experience severe, excessive sweating could be at risk for low sodium and may need special supplementation. Endurance athletes also need to replenish their electrolytes after intensive workouts when they lose a lot of fluids. People who are ill and losing high amounts of fluids through vomiting or diarrhea may need electrolyte replacement as well.

Signs of deficiency can include:

- Weakness
- Low blood pressure
- Nausea/vomiting/diarrhea
- Headaches and confusion
- Seizures
- Weight loss
- Loss of muscle function

## How Much You Need

The Dietary Guidelines for Americans recommends less than 2,300 milligrams of sodium per day, which comes out to about 1 teaspoon of salt. The American Heart Association also recommends consuming no more than 2,300 milligrams per day and, ideally, less than 1,500 milligrams of sodium per day for most adults. Your body only needs about 500 milligrams per day to function properly.

There are no specific sodium upper limits for infants, children, and teens; however certain levels of daily Adequate Intake for healthy growth have been established. These include:

| AGE | MALE | FEMALE |
| --- | --- | --- |
| 0–6 months | 110mg | 110mg |
| 7–12 months | 370mg | 370mg |
| 1–3 years | 1,000mg | 1,000mg |
| 4–8 years | 1,200mg | 1,200mg |
| 9–70 years | 1,500mg | 1,500mg |
| Pregnancy | – | 1,500mg |
| Lactation | – | 1,500mg |

### Best Way to Avoid

While most of the chapters in this book focus on how to increase your intake of certain nutrients and vitamins, sodium is an exception; in this section we'll look at how to decrease salt.

- Eat fewer highly processed foods. Start by adding 1 cup of vegetables per day instead of packaged meals or snacks. For example, if you are craving a crunchy snack, try celery and hummus instead of chips.
- Read labels and choose items that are low-sodium (140 milligrams or less per serving) or foods with no salt added.
- When eating out, ask for the dressing or sauce on the side and pair one cooked item with one raw item. For example, enjoy your burger but skip the extra sauces (like ketchup and mustard) or use less of them. Avoid the fries and add extra lettuce, tomato, and avocado to your burger instead.
- Try following the DASH diet. The Dietary Approaches to Stop Hypertension (DASH) plan has been shown to help lower blood pressure without medication. It focuses on minimizing salt and increasing foods high in potassium, calcium, and magnesium, all of which help to lower blood pressure. Emphasis is placed on eating vegetables, fruits, low-fat dairy, and some whole grains, nuts, seeds, and lean protein from fish and poultry.
- Shift toward a more plant-based or vegetarian diet.

## Food Sources

Here are the top seven sources of salt in American diets:

- Packaged/cured meats
- Burritos and tacos
- Bread and rolls
- Pizza
- Salty snacks (crackers, chips, puffs)
- Cheese/cheesy foods
- Sandwiches

| FOOD (SERVING SIZE) | SODIUM (MG) |
| --- | --- |
| Ham, roasted (3 ounces) | 1,117 |
| Shrimp, packaged, plain, frozen (3 ounces) | 800 |
| Pizza (1 large slice) | 765–957 (average amount of sodium in store-bought and frozen pizza) |
| Soup, canned (1 cup) | 700 |
| Beef jerky (1 ounce) | 620 |
| Baked beans, with sauce (½ cup) | 524 |
| Pork rinds (1 ounce) | 515 |
| Vegetable juice, packaged (8 ounces) | 405 |
| Tortillas, flour (1 round, 8 inches) | 391 |
| Processed cheese (1 slice) | 364 |
| Instant pudding mix (½ cup) | 350 |
| Vegetables (peas, asparagus), canned (½ cup) | 310–346 |
| Salad dressings (2 tablespoons) | 304 (average amount of sodium in major brand-name foods) |
| Dill pickles (1 ounce) | 241 |

# Delicious Vegan Sweet Potato Breakfast Bowl *Serves 1*

Here's an easy and delicious recipe that can help to lower sodium because it's high in potassium and magnesium. These two nutrients work together to help you balance sodium, so if you have a meal high in sodium for dinner, this could be an appropriate breakfast!

| | | |
|---|---|---|
| 1 small sweet potato | 1 tablespoon unsalted sunflower seeds | 3 tablespoons plain vegan coconut yogurt |
| 1 teaspoon ground cinnamon | 1 tablespoon chopped hazelnuts | ½ small banana, peeled |
| 1 tablespoon chopped dried apricots | | ½ tablespoon flaxseeds |
| | | ½ tablespoon chia seeds |

**PER SERVING**
*Calories: 326, Fat: 17g, Protein: 8g, Sodium: 5mg, Fiber: 13g, Carbohydrates: 42g, Sugar: 14g*

1 Preheat oven to 400°F.
2 While the oven heats, use a fork to pierce each side of potato. Wrap potato in foil, place on a baking sheet, and cook 45–60 minutes or until soft.
3 Remove potato from the oven and let cool, then slice into rounds.
4 Place the rounds in a medium bowl and add remaining ingredients. Serve immediately.

# Sulfur

Recognizable as part of the compound that gives off that terrible "rotten egg smell," sulfur isn't actually all bad. Sulfur is a macro mineral that is present throughout all of your body's tissues (it's the third-most common mineral in your system, after calcium and phosphorous). Traditionally, it hasn't been considered essential on its own, because you get most of your sulfur from certain amino acids (the building blocks of protein) in your diet. However, more recently, some researchers have hypothesized that sulfur may in fact be more important than was previously thought. It has many uses in natural medicine, as well as numerous healing, beautifying, and antimicrobial properties that are worth knowing about.

## Description

Sulfur is needed to help along some chemical reactions in the body as well as the creation of proteins, which make up muscles and tissues. It doesn't do much on its own, but as a complement to other compounds, it helps with a lot of different reactions. It's also part of one of the most important antioxidants and detoxifying compounds in your body, glutathione, as well as other enzymes and reaction catalysts that keep things like your joints, skin, hair, and nails healthy, strong, and functioning properly. Sulfur isn't usually considered essential on its own because it's part of the amino acids methionine (which is essential) and cysteine (which is conditionally essential—see the "Amino Acids, Essential" entry for more on what this means). So, if you're eating some protein-rich foods like beef, chicken, eggs, and fish, you're likely getting enough. If you don't eat meat, you can get plant-based versions of sulfur in many cruciferous veggies and foods in the allium family, like onions, garlic, shallots, and leeks.

Some hot springs contain sulfur compounds, which explains that rotten egg smell they sometimes give off. Soaking in sulfur water may help relieve some muscle pain, skin conditions, and itching— this is because sulfur is absorbed through the skin and may help slow down some of the pain receptor signals in the body. People with conditions such as arthritis may find it helpful to soak in a sulfur water bath to ease the pain.

## Role in the Body

- **Part of the body's detox system:** Sulfur helps to make up some of your liver's detoxification enzymes, which can neutralize harmful chemicals and compounds in the body.

- **Formation of proteins:** Sulfur is part of numerous proteins, such as keratin, which helps make up your nails and hair, and the amino acids methionine and cysteine, which are part of many other tissues in the body.
- **Helps to create glutathione:** As one of the key antioxidants that helps keep your cells healthy and your skin glowing, glutathione is extremely important and requires sulfur to be synthesized.

## Benefits

- **Cleansing and toxin removal:** As part of key enzymes (helpers) that help to neutralize and excrete harmful compounds, sulfur helps to detoxify your system.
- **May prevent acne and improve skin appearance:** Topically, sulfur has antibacterial effects against the bacteria that cause acne on the skin. Sulfur applied to the skin may also help with dark spots and other skin conditions.
- **May help with joint and arthritis pain:** Consuming a diet with plenty of plant-based sulfur may help relieve joint and arthritis pain. Some studies using sulfur supplements have shown a positive link between it and decreased pain.

- **Protective against cancer:** The organosulfur compounds in cruciferous vegetables are one of the main reasons foods like broccoli, Brussels sprouts, and cabbage are considered to be cancer-fighting foods.
- **Aids in protection of cells and reduction of inflammation:** As part of the super powerful antioxidant glutathione, sulfur helps it to keep cell damage and inflammation under control.
- **Helps to strengthen and maintain nails, hair, and skin:** Sufficient sulfur is needed for the formation of proteins that make up your nails, hair, and skin.

## Side Effects, Warnings, and Precautions

Sulfur from food is extremely safe, and it would be nearly impossible to get too much. Some people are likely lacking in beneficial sulfur compounds from things like cruciferous vegetables. Taking sulfur supplements, usually in the form of methylsulfonylmethane (MSM) is considered quite safe, thought taking high amounts can lead to symptoms such as diarrhea or GI discomfort.

## Signs of Deficiency

Since sulfur doesn't act alone, you need to look at the components it helps comprise to see where issues could come in with sulfur deficiency. Most of these are related to joints, tissues, and some of the detoxification enzymes.

Signs of deficiency include:

- Joint pain and disease
- Reduced production of proteins in the body
- Cell damage/reduced detoxification action

## How Much You Need

While there's no official RDA or AI for sulfur, some researchers suggest performing an analysis of "sulfur balance" in the body to determine how much you need and if you are getting enough. They have also pointed out that some segments of the population (such as the elderly) are likely not getting enough sulfur. However, more research is needed.

Other experts consider the recommendation for protein to be enough to address the need for sulfur, since it's part of the essential amino acid methionine and the conditionally essential amino acid cysteine.

No upper limit for sulfur has been established.

## Best Way to Consume

The best way to get enough sulfur is to eat a balanced diet. If you eat meat and animal products, you are almost certainly getting enough. If you are vegetarian or vegan, you may have to plan your meals a bit more carefully to include adequate cruciferous and allium vegetables to increase your sulfur intake. Depletion of nutrients in the soil can reduce the amount of sulfur absorbed into the plants. You should try to consume a serving of organic cruciferous vegetables most days and add onions and garlic when cooking your meals.

## Natural Food Sources

Foods that are high in sulfur come in two different categories:

- MSM (methylsulfonylmethane) is mostly found in plant sources such as cruciferous vegetables (cabbage, broccoli, Brussels sprouts) and allium vegetables (garlic, shallots, onions, and leeks).
- Foods high in vitamin $B_1$ (thiamin) also tend to have sulfur. Some examples include pork chops, eggs, nuts, and whole grains.

| FOOD (SERVING SIZE) | SULFUR (MG) |
| --- | --- |
| Lobster, boiled (4 ounces) | 510 |
| Crab, boiled (5 ounces) | 470 |
| Peanuts, roasted, salted (30) | 380 |

| FOOD (SERVING SIZE) | SULFUR (MG) |
|---|---|
| Dried peach (1 ounce) | 240 |
| Cod, baked (3½ ounces) | 230 |
| Cheddar cheese (1 ounce) | 230 |
| Egg, hard-boiled (1 large) | 180 |
| Almonds (10 whole) | 150 |
| Cabbage, raw (2 ounces) | 90 |
| Bran, wheat (8 grams) | 65 |
| Onion, peeled, chopped (¼ cup) | 50 |
| Barley, boiled (3½ ounces) | 35 |

## RECIPE

# Fresh and Filling Detox Bowl *Serves 1*

This bowl will support your body's natural detox system. Top with fresh cilantro for an additional flavor and detoxifying boost.

½ cup frozen riced cauliflower

1 tablespoon extra-virgin olive oil, divided

1 medium stalk spring onion, chopped

1 teaspoon turmeric

½ cup cooked barley

½ cup shredded cabbage, purple or green

¼ small avocado, peeled, pitted, and chopped

1 tablespoon grated Parmesan cheese

½ tablespoon chopped cilantro

1 tablespoon roasted pistachios

⅟₁₆ teaspoon sea salt

Pinch black pepper

**PER SERVING**
*Calories: 361, Fat: 23g, Protein: 9g, Sodium: 220mg, Fiber: 11g, Carbohydrates: 34g, Sugar: 3g*

1 In a medium skillet over medium heat, sauté cauliflower rice with half of the olive oil, the onion, and turmeric 2–3 minutes. Place into a large mixing bowl.

2 Add barley, cabbage, avocado, and remaining oil to the bowl and toss well to combine.

3 Top with Parmesan, cilantro, and pistachios.

4 Add salt and pepper as needed. Enjoy!

# Water

This nutrient may be the most important of them all. Water is the most abundant substance on planet earth, and it also happens to be the one that humans need the most of. You can last for weeks without food, but you can only survive for a few days without drinking water. Your body is 50–75 percent water. This essential nutrient has many roles and functions beyond making up a big part of your cells and organs. It helps with everything from vitamin and mineral absorption to signal transmission and waste excretion. There is conflicting information on how much water you should drink and also what kind of water—tap, bottled, the kind with minerals and special pH levels? Let's see if this entry can clear up some of the confusion.

## Description

From the beginning of time, humans evolved an extremely complex mechanism to maintain hydration. Every part of the body—from your taste buds to your kidneys—sends detailed communication signals to the brain to stimulate thirst and determine how much water to release or hold on to. Delicate adjustments are made automatically within your system, depending on how much you're losing and drinking, with your kidneys either filtering more if you are well hydrated or reabsorbing some of the fluids in your system if your body senses that you're dehydrated. Water has many special properties that make it essential to life. It's not only part of every cell; it also helps to dissolve nutrients and then transport them within your body. And, it's the ultimate detoxifier—helping to eliminate all wastes from your system.

## Role in the Body

- **Helps to keep tissues in your mouth, eyes, and nose moist:** Water is the main component of saliva, which helps to keep your mouth moist. Water also keeps all other tissues hydrated.
- **Supports regular bowel movements:** Adequate water levels are needed for stool formation and stool softening. Without enough water, foods cannot move through the intestinal tract smoothly, and this can cause constipation.
- **Dissolves minerals and vitamins to make them accessible to body tissues:** Water helps make nutrients from food more accessible to tissues.

It also aids the absorption of fiber, which boosts digestion.

- **Carries nutrients and oxygen to your cells:** Nutrients from food are carried through the body by your blood, which is 92 percent water. These nutrients are then broken down and dissolved in water.
- **Flushes bacteria away from your bladder:** Water is essential to prevent bladder infections and to maintain normal kidney function. Drinking enough water can also prevent kidney stones.
- **Aids digestion:** Water helps to break down food in all parts of the digestive tract so it can be absorbed and utilized by the body.
- **Normalizes blood pressure:** Having proper hydration helps keep your blood pressure normal.
- **Stabilizes the heartbeat:** All organs need water for normal function, and if you are dehydrated, your heart has to work harder to maintain your blood flow.
- **Cushions joints:** Joints are surrounded by water, which acts as a protective barrier.
- **Protects organs and tissues:** Water acts as a buffer to protect organs from damage.
- **Regulates body temperature:** Sweat is the body's temperature-regulation mechanism.

**Benefits**
- Boosts energy levels
- Prevents constipation
- Is a natural detoxifier
- Keeps skin and tissues hydrated, healthy, plump, and smooth
- Can prevent and treat headaches
- Helps to keep bacteria and viruses at bay
- Ensures a stable heartbeat and body temperature
- Optimizes nutrition and digestion
- Helps with weight loss and weight management
- Improves sports and athletic performance

**Side Effects, Warnings, and Precautions**

Water has zero side effects when you drink it in normal and adequate amounts. If you drink a lot of water quickly, you may feel the uncomfortable urge to urinate come on quickly. In really extreme cases, drinking a huge amount of water can lead to a very dangerous condition called hyponatremia, which throws off the balance of electrolytes (sodium) inside your body. This is very rare and only a concern if you consume massive quantities of water in a short time (2–6 gallons over a period of a few hours). People with heart conditions, high blood pressure, and kidney problems may need to be careful to not drink too much water.

## Signs of Deficiency

As we get older, our natural thirst mechanisms start to get a little bit blunted, so we may not feel thirst as quickly, which is why older adults are at a higher risk of dehydration. Infants and young children are also more sensitive to fluid shifts. Those with certain chronic conditions like diabetes and people who lose a lot of sweat due to heavy workouts can also be at risk.

Signs of deficiency (dehydration) can include:

- Thirst and dry mouth
- Less frequent urination and very dark-colored urine
- Constipation
- Headaches
- Muscle cramps
- Irritability
- Dizziness
- Sunken eyes

## How Much You Need

There's actually no specific rule on how much water you should drink; this is determined by many factors, such as your environment, how much you're losing via sweat and other bodily fluids, as well as your nutrient levels and even body temperature. The Institute of Medicine of the National Academies recommends that while people should let their thirst guide their fluid intake, women should aim for 2.7 liters (91 ounces) of total water each day, and men should aim for 3.7 liters (125 ounces). These numbers take into account both food and liquid sources. The Adequate Intake for total water (liters per day) is:

| AGE | MALE | FEMALE |
| --- | --- | --- |
| 0–6 months | 0.7 L/d | 0.7 L/d |
| 7–12 months | 0.8 L/d | 0.8 L/d |
| 1–3 years | 1.3 L/d | 1.3 L/d |
| 4–8 years | 1.7 L/d | 1.7 L/d |
| 9–13 years | 2.4 L/d | 2.1 L/d |
| 14–18 years | 3.3 L/d | 2.3 L/d |
| 19–69 years | 3.7 L/d | 2.7 L/d |
| 70+ years | 3.7 L/d | 2.7 L/d |
| Pregnancy | – | 3.0 L/d |
| Lactation | – | 3.8 L/d |

## Best Way to Consume

There's a lot of confusion and myths about the best kinds and sources of water. Let's review the most common ones:

- **Bottled is better:** Wrong! Almost all water systems in the US are treated and filtered. You can get a filter system for your home to clean the water even further and improve the taste.

Plus, plastic bottles are terrible for the environment and recent studies show that some of the plastic leaches into the water as well.

- **Alkaline water is more beneficial:** This is a myth, but a lot of companies are making a lot of money by promoting "pH-balanced water." Your body has its own tightly regulated pH-balancing system, and alkaline water is unlikely to affect this in any way.
- **Filtered water is necessary:** This is a matter of preference, not a necessity. If you find you like the taste of filtered water, try a reverse osmosis or ceramic gravity filter. You can also use a basic counter filter.
- **Using your own refillable container is dirty and gross due to bacterial buildup:** False. Try getting a stainless steel reusable bottle or glass bottle and use it only for water. You can rinse it with soapy water every couple of days, and there will be no problems with contamination.

## Natural Food Sources

| FOOD (SERVING SIZE) | WATER % OF FOOD WEIGHT |
|---|---|
| Lettuce, green leaf (1 cup) | 95% |
| Celery, raw (1 medium stalk) | 95% |
| Tomato, raw, chopped (½ cup) | 94% |
| Cantaloupe, chopped (1 cup) | 90% |
| Broccoli, raw, chopped (½ cup) | 89% |
| Orange juice (½ cup) | 89% |
| Grapefruit, white (½ medium) | 88% |
| Potato, white, baked with skin (1 medium) | 75% |
| Pasta, boiled (¾ cup) | 72% |
| Ground beef, hot dogs, tenderloin steak (3 ounces) | 50–59% |
| Pizza (1 slice) | 40–49% |
| Bagel (1 medium), or bread (1 slice) | 30–39% |
| Butter, margarine (1 tablespoon) | 10–19% |

# Hydrating Summer Salad *Serves 2*

This fresh and fun salad is packed with high-water foods. It's perfect for summer parties and helps you stay hydrated by adding a lot of water from foods to your diet.

| | | |
|---|---|---|
| 2 cups chopped romaine lettuce | ¼ cup crumbled feta cheese | 1 tablespoon balsamic vinegar |
| 1 Persian cucumber, chopped | 1 tablespoon slivered roasted almonds | 1 teaspoon dried oregano |
| 2 cups watermelon cubes | 2 tablespoons extra-virgin olive oil | Pinch salt |
| | | Pinch black pepper |

**PER SERVING**

*Calories: 271, Fat: 19g, Protein: 6g, Sodium: 326mg, Fiber: 3g, Carbohydrates: 22g, Sugar: 15g, Water: 344g*

1 Combine lettuce, cucumber, watermelon, feta cheese, and almonds in a medium bowl.

2 In a small bowl, combine the oil, vinegar, oregano, salt, and pepper to make a dressing. Drizzle dressing over salad to your liking and enjoy.

# Zinc

When was the last time you thought about how extraordinary your senses of smell and taste are? Probably our most underappreciated sense, our ability to smell is one of our most powerful, primitive senses and is closely linked to memory and emotion. Zinc is a trace mineral that is essential for these senses. It's also needed for a huge number of other vital functions and processes in your body, ranging from wound healing to replication of genetic material. It's vital to ensure that you're consuming sufficient zinc—and many people are not. In this entry you'll learn about the best ways to obtain zinc from the foods you eat and the numerous benefits associated with it.

## Description

Worldwide, zinc is one of the most prevalent micronutrient deficiencies, alongside vitamin A, iron, and iodine. The World Health Organization has cited zinc deficiency as a significant global nutrition issue, with about one third of people globally likely to have inadequate intakes.

Why is zinc so important? It is essential for your immune health and necessary for wound healing. It can be beneficial for gut health as well. One study done in India showed that zinc can reduce the frequency and duration of diarrhea episodes in children. This is important because lack of clean water and poor sanitation lead to diarrhea, which can quickly progress to malnutrition in very young children. So, adequate zinc intake may help to alleviate one of the major underlying causes of malnutrition in kids globally. In addition, about 250 different proteins in the body have zinc, many of which make up enzymes, or helper molecules, to create and replicate your genes.

## Role in the Body

- **Essential for smell and taste receptors:** One of the compounds necessary for your senses of smell and taste is dependent on zinc for its functioning.
- **Critical for more than one hundred enzyme systems in the body:** Enzymes play a key role in cellular functions throughout the body. Some key systems include those related to maintaining water and electrolyte balance, blood pressure, and metabolism.
- **Regulates nucleoproteins:** Zinc is important in the process of how DNA helps create proteins essential for body functions.
- **Regulates inflammatory cells:** Zinc is involved in triggering activation of inflammatory pathways in cells.

- **Important factor in growth, tissue repair, and wound healing:** This mineral is a part of almost all the systems that help to heal, repair, and create new tissues after an injury or burn.
- **Helps regulate immune response:** Zinc is involved in the function of immune cells such as phagocytes and T-cells, which are essential to a healthy immune system for fighting off infections.
- **Important for male health:** Zinc helps produce hormones such as testosterone and can help to increase sperm count.
- **May inhibit effects of infections:** Zinc may help to prevent pathogens like *E. coli* and cholera from infecting the body.

## Benefits

- Well-functioning immune system
- Faster wound healing
- May shorten the duration of colds
- Needed for senses of smell and taste
- Smooth replication and repair of DNA
- Proper growth in childhood
- May improve fertility

## Side Effects, Warnings, and Precautions

Getting zinc from food sources won't cause any adverse reactions or symptoms. However, zinc supplements can cause side effects such as nausea, vomiting, stomach cramps, diarrhea, and headaches. Over time, taking too much supplemental zinc can cause copper deficiency, as these minerals compete for absorption in the body. Zinc supplements may also interact with some medications like antibiotics. Talk to your doctor before starting any supplements if you have medical conditions or are on any medications. An additional word of caution: Avoid nasal spray or gel with zinc; these products have been linked to total loss of smell.

## Signs of Deficiency

As mentioned, low intake of zinc is a significant issue worldwide. People who are vegan or vegetarian need to be particularly careful to eat foods with enough zinc, because it is higher in animal products, and while there are plant-based sources, it tends to be less bioavailable (not absorbed as well) in these foods. A very rare genetic condition called acrodermatitis enteropathica causes problems with zinc absorption, but this can be treated with high-dose supplements.

Signs of deficiency can include:

- Poor wound healing
- Diarrhea
- Eye and skin problems
- Impairments in the senses of smell and taste
- Thinning hair and hair loss

- Poor appetite
- Poor growth and stunting
- Problems with reproductive organs

## How Much You Need

Everything but 0–6 month amounts are in RDA.

| AGE | MALE | FEMALE |
|---|---|---|
| 0–6 months | 2mg (AI) | 2mg (AI) |
| 7–12 months | 3mg | 3mg |
| 1–3 years | 3mg | 3mg |
| 4–8 years | 5mg | 5mg |
| 9–13 years | 8mg | 8mg |
| 14–18 years | 11mg | 9mg |
| 19+ years | 11mg | 8mg |
| Pregnancy | – | 11mg |
| Lactation | – | 12mg |

## Upper Limits (Amount Per Day)

| AGE | MALE | FEMALE |
|---|---|---|
| 0–6 months | 4mg | 4mg |
| 7–12 months | 5mg | 5mg |
| 1–3 years | 7mg | 7mg |
| 4–8 years | 12mg | 12mg |
| 9–13 years | 23mg | 23mg |
| 14–18 years | 34mg | 34mg |
| 19+ years | 40mg | 40mg |
| Pregnancy | – | 40mg |
| Lactation | – | 40mg |

## Best Way to Consume

Zinc is highest in animal products and is best absorbed from these products. Some plant-based foods contain some zinc, but they can also contain other substances that inhibit the absorption of this mineral. Oysters have more zinc than any other food, by far! Vegans will need to carefully plan out their meals to make sure they are getting enough zinc. If you aren't sure whether you're meeting your needs, especially if you follow a plant-based diet, meet with a dietitian to help you optimize your intake and make sure you're getting enough.

## Natural Food Sources

| FOOD (SERVING SIZE) | ZINC (MG) |
|---|---|
| Oyster, breaded and fried (3 ounces) | 74 |
| Liver, veal, cooked (2½ ounces) | 8.4–8.9 |
| Beef chuck, braised (3 ounces) | 7 |
| Lobster, cooked (3 ounces) | 3.4 |

| FOOD (SERVING SIZE) | ZINC (MG) |
| --- | --- |
| Dark chocolate, 70%–80% (3½ ounces) | 3.3 |
| Pumpkin seeds, dried (1 ounce) | 2.2 |
| Lentils, cooked (¾ cup) | 1.9 |
| Ricotta cheese (½ cup) | 1.8 |
| Cashews, dry roasted (1 ounce) | 1.6 |
| Oatmeal, plain, prepared with water (1 packet) | 1.1 |
| Milk, low-fat (1 cup) | 1 |
| Kidney beans, cooked (½ cup) | 0.9 |

## RECIPE

# Beef and Veggie Chili *Serves 2*

This chili is comforting and healthy at the same time. You can even add some more vege-tables in this chili to add more nutrients and flavor. Enjoy with some shredded cheese or salsa on top, and serve with a side of whole-grain bread to round out the meal.

| | | |
| --- | --- | --- |
| 2 tablespoons avocado oil | ½ cup lentils, cooked | Pinch black pepper |
| 1 small onion, peeled and chopped | ½ (16-ounce) can lima beans, drained | 2 cups low-sodium beef broth |
| 8 ounces ground beef | ½ teaspoon cayenne pepper | 1 cup canned, no-salt-added diced tomatoes |
| 1 medium carrot, diced | 1 teaspoon cumin | 2 tablespoons tomato paste |
| ¼ cup corn kernels | 1/16 teaspoon salt | |

**PER SERVING**
*Calories: 618, Fat: 29g, Protein: 36g, Sodium: 614mg, Fiber: 13g, Carbohydrates: 47g, Sugar: 10g, Zinc: 6.8mg*

1 Heat oil in a large stockpot over medium heat. Add onions and cook until softened. Add beef and cook 5–7 minutes.

2 Add carrots, corn, lentils, beans, cayenne, cumin, salt, and pepper and combine well. Cook 3 minutes.

3 Add broth, diced tomatoes, and tomato paste. Simmer for another 20–30 minutes, then serve.

# Vitamin Z, Sleep

Have you heard of vitamin Z? It's one that a lot of people aren't getting enough of—sleep. Sleep is essential for health and disease prevention. Despite very strong evidence proving the importance of sleep, many health professionals often fail to emphasize the role of this important health behavior. Sleep duration, as well as quality and timing, can determine how well your body regulates your metabolism and manages emotions. It can also determine how well you perform physically and mentally and how fast you learn new skills. Sleep is as important as a balanced diet or physical activity in maintaining health and weight.

## Description

Nutrition and sleep are closely linked. Your sleep affects certain hormone levels that impact your hunger and fullness signals. Have you ever noticed that you are hungrier and eat more when you are sleep-deprived? That's thanks to a hormone called ghrelin, which stimulates hunger and appetite and increases when you don't get enough sleep. There are also different foods and beverages as well as ways to eat and drink them that can impact your sleep.

Just as essential as breathing and eating, sleep is part of the framework for optimal health. Driving a car while sleep-deprived can be just as dangerous as driving drunk. Deficiency can also lead to all kinds of physical and mental problems, from heart disease to depression to impaired immunity. Sleep is included in this book because it is so vitally important to your health.

## Role in the Body

- **Hormone regulation:** Sleep affects many different hormone levels, but two of the key ones are called leptin and ghrelin, which affect hunger and fullness signals. When you get adequate sleep, levels of leptin increase, helping you feel less hungry. With insufficient sleep, your levels of ghrelin rise and make you feel hungrier.
- **Support of the immune system:** The entire immune system depends on sleep to function properly. With lack of sleep you can become more susceptible to infections and illness.
- **Healing and repair of tissues and vessels:** When you are in a deep state of sleep, this releases a hormone that helps to repair cells in the body.

- **Muscle growth:** Sleep also triggers hormones that promote growth and muscle mass.
- **Insulin utilization:** Insulin is the hormone that signals your cells to take in sugar from the blood. Getting enough sleep helps to ensure that insulin is used properly. Not getting adequate sleep can cause elevated blood sugar levels.
- **Healthy weight:** Numerous studies have shown that not getting enough sleep increases the risk of weight gain and obesity.
- **Formation of new pathways in the brain that help you learn and memorize:** Scientists have found that some brain cells actually begin to fire differently during sleep and the connections between different cell networks are developed during this time, imprinting memories and information.

## Benefits

- Improved memory and learning ability
- Healthier weight due to well-balanced hormones
- Improved mood and feelings of well-being
- Decreased risk of heart disease
- Stronger immune system
- Fewer cravings
- Improved memory and learning
- Healthier blood sugar levels

## Side Effects, Warnings, and Precautions

Getting less sleep than your body needs can affect all areas of your life: your work, exercise, driving, social skills, and, of course, your diet and health. Different age groups need different amounts of sleep. The recommended range is seven to nine hours for most adults. Very few people can function optimally on less than this, though many think they can! Lack of sleep can lead to a lot of health problems, such as weight gain, heart disease, high blood sugar, depression, and more.

## Signs of Deficiency

While sleep deficiency can affect anyone, certain groups of people are more at risk. This includes people who work late-night or erratic shifts at work, like healthcare workers and travelers. People who drink alcohol or take drugs will have disrupted sleep cycles. Some medical issues like anxiety, depression, and sleep disorders will also interfere with sleep.

Signs of deficiency can include:

- Fatigue
- Increased food cravings
- Irritability
- Trouble concentrating and remembering information
- Mood swings
- Increased anxiety

- Weight gain
- Elevated blood sugar
- Increased risk of accidents

## How Much You Need

The National Sleep Foundation (NSF), along with a multidisciplinary expert panel, issued its new recommendations for appropriate sleep durations:

| AGE | MALE | FEMALE |
| --- | --- | --- |
| 0–3 months | 14–17 hours | 14–17 hours |
| 4–11 months | 12–15 hours | 12–15 hours |
| 1–2 years | 11–14 hours | 11–14 hours |
| 3–5 years | 10–13 hours | 10–13 hours |
| 6–13 years | 9–11 hours | 9–11 hours |
| 14–17 years | 8–10 hours | 8–10 hours |
| 18–25 years | 7–9 hours | 7–9 hours |
| 26–64 years | 7–9 hours | 7–9 hours |
| 65+ years | 7–8 hours | 7–8 hours |

## Best Way to Optimize Sleep

There are many things you can do nutrition- and food-wise to help you sleep better. Here are some tips for how and when to eat and drink so that you can optimize your vitamin Z!

- Avoid caffeine for six to eight hours before bedtime.
- Avoid alcohol for three to four hours before bedtime.
- A small serving of carbs (about ½ cup) can help some people get to sleep.

- Exercise during the day will help you rest at night (but not less than two hours before bedtime, as it may keep you revved up and awake).
- Warm milk or yogurt before bed may help you go to sleep, but this is linked more to the comforting feeling versus the tryptophan levels (which are likely too low to have much of an impact).
- Soothing herbal teas such as chamomile and lavender have been shown to help promote relaxation and sleep.

**Natural Food Sources That May Help with Sleep**

- Almonds, 1 small handful
- Banana, peeled, 1 medium
- Chicken, 2–3 ounces
- Chamomile tea, 1 cup
- Cottage cheese, ½ cup
- Egg, 1 large
- Honey, 1 tablespoon
- Kale, 1 cup
- Kiwi, 1 medium
- Oatmeal, cooked, ½ cup
- Passion flower tea, 1 cup
- Peppermint tea, 1 cup
- Prunes, 2–3
- Tart cherry juice, ½ cup
- Warm milk, ½ cup
- Yogurt, ½ cup

## RECIPE

# Sleepy Time Oatmeal  *Serves 1*

In addition to the toppings listed in this recipe, feel free to add more, such as ¼ cup sliced banana, kiwi, nuts, or a sprinkle of cinnamon.

| | | |
|---|---|---|
| ½ cup old-fashioned oats | 1 tablespoon dried cherries | 1 tablespoon cottage cheese |
| ½ cup low-fat milk | | ½ teaspoon honey |

**PER SERVING**
*Calories: 263, Fat: 4g, Protein: 11g, Sodium: 105mg, Fiber: 5g, Carbohydrates: 47g, Sugar: 11g*

1  In a small saucepan over medium heat, cook oats in milk until milk is fully absorbed, about 5 minutes.
2  Add cherries and stir to combine.
3  Top with cottage cheese and honey and enjoy!

# Final Thoughts

As a dietitian, entrepreneur, and humanitarian, I have a unique perspective on health, nutrition, and sustainability. My family came to the US from the former Soviet Union when I was seven years old, as political refugees. Growing up, I loved the traditional Russian and Ukrainian dishes that my mom would make, like the quintessential beetroot soup, borscht; golubtsi (stuffed cabbage leaves); and grechka (buckwheat). I also came to love American food—everything from mac 'n' cheese to pumpkin pie (which my Russian family always found very strange). My fascination with food and nutrition grew as I began to love travel and discovering different dishes and cuisines.

After finishing my registered dietitian nutritionist and master of public health degrees, I pursued my dream of working internationally in development and humanitarian aid. I spent two years with an international NGO in Geneva, Switzerland, and then five years in Africa, where my work was mainly focused on the treatment and prevention of severe acute malnutrition in children and women.

My time in Africa, where I worked in Gabon, Ethiopia, Sudan, South Sudan, and Chad, transformed my life and outlook on the world, and helped me to realize both how very fortunate we are and also the tremendous responsibility that we each have to give back. It also reminded me how interconnected we are, both with one another and our planet.

Watching climate change decimate the livelihoods of subsistence farmers in places like Ethiopia and Chad was the catalyst for my passion for the environment. I returned to L.A. and launched my brand and private practice, Nomadista Nutrition, as well as an innovative food product, Mini Fish, which you can learn more about at minifish.co.

People ask me all the time how I eat. My eating is informed by my background, scientific knowledge, and commitment to sustainability. With over seven billion mouths to feed, we must consider the implications of our food choices more than ever before. Due to the environmental and ethical impacts of animal agriculture, I have reduced my consumption of animal products—and I no longer eat beef, the worst offender. I strive to consume more plant-based foods than not, but I do eat animal protein regularly, with a heavier focus on sustainable seafood. I love coffee and chocolate and have both pretty much daily. Doughnuts are my "guilty pleasure" but I don't feel guilty when I eat them—I believe that indulgences are part of a healthy diet and happy life.

After working all over the world—from top medical centers in the US to tiny villages in rural Africa, I can confidently say that there is no shortcut to good health. But, there are some fundamental practices that you can incorporate into your lifestyle, no matter how busy you are. Hopefully you have found this book helpful to understanding how to nourish your body, optimize your well-being, and, best of all, fully enjoy getting your nutrients and vitamins by eating delicious (and real) food.

# US/Metric Conversion Charts

## VOLUME CONVERSIONS

| US VOLUME MEASURE | METRIC EQUIVALENT |
| --- | --- |
| 1/8 teaspoon | 0.5 milliliter |
| 1/4 teaspoon | 1 milliliter |
| 1/2 teaspoon | 2 milliliters |
| 1 teaspoon | 5 milliliters |
| 1/2 tablespoon | 7 milliliters |
| 1 tablespoon (3 teaspoons) | 15 milliliters |
| 2 tablespoons (1 fluid ounce) | 30 milliliters |
| 1/4 cup (4 tablespoons) | 60 milliliters |
| 1/3 cup | 90 milliliters |
| 1/2 cup (4 fluid ounces) | 125 milliliters |
| 2/3 cup | 160 milliliters |
| 3/4 cup (6 fluid ounces) | 180 milliliters |
| 1 cup (16 tablespoons) | 250 milliliters |
| 1 pint (2 cups) | 500 milliliters |
| 1 quart (4 cups) | 1 liter (about) |

## WEIGHT CONVERSIONS

| US WEIGHT MEASURE | METRIC EQUIVALENT |
| --- | --- |
| 1/2 ounce | 15 grams |
| 1 ounce | 30 grams |
| 2 ounces | 60 grams |
| 3 ounces | 85 grams |
| 1/4 pound (4 ounces) | 115 grams |
| 1/2 pound (8 ounces) | 225 grams |
| 3/4 pound (12 ounces) | 340 grams |
| 1 pound (16 ounces) | 454 grams |

## OVEN TEMPERATURE CONVERSIONS

| DEGREES FAHRENHEIT | DEGREES CELSIUS |
|---|---|
| 200 degrees F | 95 degrees C |
| 250 degrees F | 120 degrees C |
| 275 degrees F | 135 degrees C |
| 300 degrees F | 150 degrees C |
| 325 degrees F | 160 degrees C |
| 350 degrees F | 180 degrees C |
| 375 degrees F | 190 degrees C |
| 400 degrees F | 205 degrees C |
| 425 degrees F | 220 degrees C |
| 450 degrees F | 230 degrees C |

## BAKING PAN SIZES

| AMERICAN | METRIC |
|---|---|
| 8 × 1½ inch round baking pan | 20 × 4 cm cake tin |
| 9 × 1½ inch round baking pan | 23 × 3.5 cm cake tin |
| 11 × 7 × 1½ inch baking pan | 28 × 18 × 4 cm baking tin |
| 13 × 9 × 2 inch baking pan | 30 × 20 × 5 cm baking tin |
| 2 quart rectangular baking dish | 30 × 20 × 3 cm baking tin |
| 15 × 10 × 2 inch baking pan | 30 × 25 × 2 cm baking tin (Swiss roll tin) |
| 9 inch pie plate | 22 × 4 or 23 × 4 cm pie plate |
| 7 or 8 inch springform pan | 18 or 20 cm springform or loose bottom cake tin |
| 9 × 5 × 3 inch loaf pan | 23 × 13 × 7 cm or 2 lb narrow loaf or pâté tin |
| 1½ quart casserole | 1.5 liter casserole |
| 2 quart casserole | 2 liter casserole |

# Index

Bowls—*continued*
Low-Carb Asian Rice Bowl, *88*
Perfect Probiotic Breakfast Bowl, *170*
Rice Bowl with Kimchi and Natto, *120*
Sushi Rice Bowl with Wild Rice, *73*
Wild Rice Detox Bowl, *56*
Brain development, 52, 74, 107, 141
Brain health, 53, 141. *See also* Alzheimer's
disease and dementia
Broccoli, recipes with, *24, 81, 116*
Bulgur, in Green Bulgur Bowl, *130*

**C**
Calcium, 65–*69*, 89, 90, 91, 117, 118, 122,
128, 148, 149, 164, 175
Cancer and cancer risk
antioxidants and, 25, 26–27
calcium and, 66
fiber and, 99
fluoride and, 93, 94
folate and, 53, 58
molybdenum and, 137
omega-3s and, 141
omega-6s and, 146
polyphenols and, 153
probiotics and, 168
selenium and, 171, 172
sulfur and, 181
vitamin A and, 10
vitamin C and, 62
vitamin D and, 89
vitamin E and, 94
Carbohydrates, processing, 122–23
Cauliflower rice, *88, 102, 183*
Cell repair and maintenance, 19
Cell structure and communication, 10, 74, 94
Cherry Chocolate Peanut Polyphenol Boost Bowl,
*157*
Chicken

Hummus Baked Chicken with Quinoa and
Zucchini, *23*
Kale Salad with Chicken, *40*
Salsa and Lime Chicken Tacos, *152*
Chili, beef and veggie, *192*
Chloride, 70–*73*
Chocolate
Cherry Chocolate Peanut Polyphenol Boost
Bowl, *157*
Chocolate Pecan Prebiotic Smoothie, *166*
Dark Chocolate Mousse with Blueberries and
Strawberries, *29*
Cholesterol production and levels, 37, 41, 42,
93–94, 98, 99, 168
Choline, 74–*77*
Chromium, 78–*81*
Cobalt, 82–*84*
Coconut, in Peachy Keen Coconut Smoothie, *135*
Collagen formation, 61, 85, 112, 127, 128
Colorful Chromium-Rich Chickpea Salad with
Broccoli, *81*
Copper, 85–*88*
Cramps, muscle, 66, 127

**D**
Dark Chocolate Mousse with Blueberries and
Strawberries, *29*
Delicious Vegan Sweet Potato Breakfast Bowl,
*179*
Dementia. *See* Alzheimer's disease and dementia
Depression, 20, 45, 53, 57, 58, 90, 94, 123, 141,
168, 194
Detoxing. *See* Toxins and detoxification
Diabetes, 31, 32, 38, 66, 78, 80, 145, 154.
*See also* Blood sugar levels; Insulin
Digestion, aiding. *See also* Probiotics
chloride, stomach acid and, 70
enzyme creation and, 19
fiber and, 98, 99